Caring For People With Alzheimer's Disease:

A Manual For Facility Staff
Second Edition

by Lisa P. Gwyther

Associate Clinical Professor
Department of Psychiatry and Behavioral Sciences
Duke University Medical Center
Durham, North Carolina

Prepared as a joint venture between the
American Health Care Association
and the
Alzheimer's Association

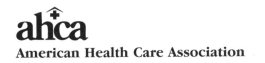

American Health Care Association

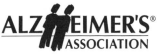

Someone to Stand by You

Staff:
Paul Stearns, Manager, Performance Measurement, Quality Improvement, American Health Care Association
Julie Dolci, Specialist, Program Services Division, Alzheimer's Association
Marla Fern Gold, Editor, Project Manager
Lynda Grahill, Copy Editor

American Health Care Association
1201 L Street, N.W.
Washington, D.C. 20005
www.ahca.org

Alzheimer's Association
919 N. Michigan Ave., Suite 1100
Chicago, Illinois 60611-1676
www.alz.org

Library of Congress Cataloging-in-Publication Data

Gwyther, Lisa P.
 Caring for people with Alzheimer's disease: a manual for facility staff / by Lisa P. Gwyther; prepared as a joint venture between the American Health Care Association and the Alzheimer's Association staff.– 2nd ed.
      p. cm.
Includes bibliographical references and index.
 ISBN 0-9705219-3-6 (alk. paper)
1. Alzheimer's disease–Nursing–Handbooks, manuals, etc. 2. Alzheimer's disease–Patients–Rehabilitation–Handbooks, manuals, etc.
I. American Health Care Association. II. Alzheimer's Association.
III. Title.
 RC523 .G88 2001
 616.8'31–dc21

                                                           2001000090

01 02 03 04 05 / 5 4 3 2 1

Caring For People With Alzheimer's Disease:

A Manual For Facility Staff
Second Edition

by Lisa P. Gwyther

TABLE OF CONTENTS

FOREWORD

The Alzheimer's Association joins the American Health Care Association (AHCA) to promote state-of-the-art, compassionate caregiving for people with Alzheimer's disease and related memory disorders. Sixteen years ago, AHCA and the Alzheimer's Association published *Care of Alzheimer's Patients: A Manual for Nursing Home Staff*. With publication of this second edition, these organizations have updated this original and popular book.

Researchers know more today about memory disorders and how to respond to residents and their families. Today, caregivers, designers, activities staff, and behavioral experts have more experience in creating special environments, activities, policies, and procedures using a "person-centered" care philosophy that better meets both the needs of residents with Alzheimer's disease and the expectations of their families.

The Alzheimer's Association is the premier source of information and support for the 4 million Americans with Alzheimer's disease. Through its national network of chapters, it offers a broad range of programs and services for people with the disease, their families, and caregivers, and represents their interests on Alzheimer-related issues before federal, state, and local governments and with health and long term care providers. The largest private funder of Alzheimer research, the Association has committed more than $100 million toward research into the causes, treatment, prevention, and cure of Alzheimer's disease.

AHCA is a nationwide federation of affiliated health care associations, together representing more than 12,000 nonprofit and for-profit assisted living and nursing facility providers, subacute care providers, and intermediate care facilities for the mentally retarded. Together, these facilities care for more than 1 million elderly and disabled individuals nationally. AHCA supports and models supportive environments where professional and compassionate care is delivered in safe and secure settings. Through its national network, AHCA works to ensure access to long term care.

AHCA and the Alzheimer's Association extend a sincere thank you to author Lisa P. Gwyther, a social worker, associate clinical professor in the Department of Psychiatry and Behavioral Sciences at Duke University Medical Center, and Senior Fellow of the Duke University Center for Aging in Durham, N.C. Ms. Gwyther has 30 years of experience in Alzheimer's services and directs Duke University's Family Support Program, a state clearinghouse, training, and information center for families and professionals caring for people with Alzheimer's. In 1999, Duke's Family Support Program was named the Agency of the Year by the National Association of Social Workers, North Carolina Chapter. Ms. Gwyther also directs education for the Bryan Alzheimer's Disease Research Center at Duke and is on the faculty of Duke's Institute on Care at the End of Life. She has published extensively on Alzheimer's residential care and is the author of the first edition of this book.

The Associations also wish to thank the reviewers, who provided valuable expertise during the revision of this book:

Melanie Chavin
Greater Chicagoland Chapter
of the Alzheimer's Association
Skokie, Illinois

Sam Fazio
Alzheimer's Association
Chicago, Illinois

Sandra Fitzler
American Health Care
Association
Washington, D.C.

Patricia E. Harkey
Sisters of Charity/Marian Hall
Mt. Carmel
Dubuque, Iowa

Carly R. Hellen
Enterprises, Inc.
Deerfield, Illinois

Sheryl Ludeke-Smith
American Retirement Corp.
Brentwood, Tennessee

Katie Maslow
Alzheimer's Association
Washington, D.C.

Diane M. Overturf
Sisters of Charity/Marian Hall
Mt. Carmel
Dubuque, Iowa

Sherry Reid
HCR-Manor Care
Toledo, Ohio

Jana Richmond
Alterra Healthcare
Molalla, Oregon

Beverly Sanborn
Senior Living Services,
Marriott International
Washington, D.C.

Cheryl Siefert
Rocky Mountain Chapter of the
Alzheimer's Association
Denver, Colorado

Sara Sinclair
Sunshine Terrace Foundation, Inc.
Logan, Utah

Eric G. Tangalos, M.D.
Mayo Clinic
Rochester, Minnesota

David Troxel
Santa Barbara Chapter of the
Alzheimer's Association
Santa Barbara, California

Tal B. Widdes
Senior Living Services,
Marriott International
Washington, D.C.

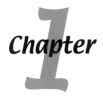

Chapter

INTRODUCTION

'Whether it afflicts a neighbor who quietly fades behind the upstairs curtains, a relative who no longer comes to visit during the holidays, or a former president, the effects of Alzheimer's disease are drawing closer to each of us every day.'

—Maureen Reagan, daughter of former President Ronald Reagan (who has Alzheimer's disease), in testimony to the House Appropriations Committee, April 15, 1999

More than 70 percent of the 2 million residents of nursing facilities, and 30 percent of people living in assisted living and other residential settings, have Alzheimer's disease (AD) or a related memory disorder. Residents with Alzheimer's share a wide range of sometimes challenging behaviors, such as aggression, agitation, eating problems, delusions, excessive worry, disinterest, pacing, and withdrawal. As a result, caring for these residents requires a lot of skill, patience, and knowledge.

Caregivers need to know there are treatments available to help residents with AD live with their illness, and much can be done in the residential or long term care facility environment to preserve dignity and quality of life for these individuals. The goal of this book is to make sense of Alzheimer care in the full range of residential facilities where people with Alzheimer's live.

Is This Book For Me?

- Do you care for people with Alzheimer's disease, such as in an assisted living or nursing facility setting?
- Did you ever wonder what it might feel like to have AD or a related disorder?
- Could you use help understanding why residents with Alzheimer's or other memory disorders think, talk, or behave the way they do?
- Could you use some fresh, practical ideas for comforting and helping residents with AD?
- Are you pressed for time by the demands of your job?
- Is your job stressful?
- Do you have no time for lectures, books, conferences, or in-service training?

If you answered "yes" to any of these questions, this book is for you.

Anyone who works directly with people with AD or other memory disorders knows that life is not easy for people with Alzheimer's, their caregivers, or their families. People with Alzheimer's are looking for something familiar—some security in a world that no longer makes sense. Increasingly, families are looking for that security in a long term care or assisted living facility. Families are looking for reassurance that staff will treat "mother" as they do and understand the pain and anguish the family is experiencing. This book addresses those needs.

Person-Centered Care

The stories and strategies provided within these pages should increase caregivers' capacity, confidence, and satisfaction with their work. The person-centered communication, activity, and environmental tips provided can help to increase the comfort and decrease the distress and fear that contribute to behavioral symptoms of Alzheimer's disease. Caregivers most likely will recognize parts of people they have known and worked with in the stories.

Everyone who works in residential or nursing facility settings cares or will care for people with AD or related disorders because the number of people diagnosed with Alzheimer's is growing every year. Facility staff are recognizing the need to know more about Alzheimer care because they, too, have family members living with this disease. Whether you are an experienced facility staff member, a family member of someone with Alzheimer's, or new to Alzheimer care, we hope this book will help you respond to the behavioral and communication challenges that occur with AD.

How To Use This Book

The following chapter provides an update of what happens to the brain of an individual with AD or a related disorder. Different types of dementias are explored and current treatments are outlined.

Chapter Three is the heart of this book. This chapter provides no-nonsense, practical suggestions for creating positive caregiving moments with AD residents and their families. Each scenario illustrates a behavioral symptom or challenge common to Alzheimer's care. For each major behavioral symptom or sign, strategies are listed that encompass tips for communication and performing activities of daily living (ADLs), activities programming, and modifying the resident's environment to minimize unwanted effects on the resident, staff, family, and other residents of the facility.

Chapter Four presents specific tools and recommendations to help families transition to long term care placement. The chapter provides an ideal family-centered approach—from admission through ongoing care.

Chapter Five offers ideas for creating special environments that make "sense" to a person with Alzheimer's, from small group settings to creating mock neighborhoods that reflect residents' "reality."

Chapter Six is for you, the caregiver, with tips on what to do when you are having a rough day. Finally, the **Appendices** provide resources for new staff or for in-service training and list contact information for organizations, Web sites, publications, and other resources that offer in-depth information on Alzheimer's care.

This book can be reviewed in sections. Start with what you need to know now and review other issues as they come up. Most importantly, do not become overwhelmed by the lists of caregiving suggestions. Try one idea at a time until you develop a collection of techniques that work for you.

Chapter 2

WHAT HAPPENS WHEN A PERSON HAS ALZHEIMER'S DISEASE?

'It's like being on an island in the middle of the ocean. I can't see land. I don't know if anyone knows I'm here or will come for me. I don't know where my next meal will come from or where I will sleep tonight.'

—*Resident with Alzheimer's*

Alzheimer's disease develops slowly and causes changes in the brain long before there are obvious changes in a person's memory, thinking, use of words, or behavior. People who experience changes in memory but can still function on their own are said to have "mild cognitive impairment" or preclinical Alzheimer's disease. Many of these people will develop Alzheimer's in three to five years. Even when loss of recent memory is obvious, people in the early stages of Alzheimer's generally look and feel the same as they did before the onset of symptoms.

AD is common in older people but it is not a normal part of growing old. It is a brain disease that causes measurable changes in the size of the brain and the way the brain uses energy and sends messages. The brains of people with Alzheimer's do not work like the brains of people without AD, or even like the brain did before the person developed Alzheimer's. Everyone with Alzheimer's loses abilities in ways that make it impossible to do things they did before, whether it was keeping house or running a business.

People with AD generally have trouble with new learning, and practicing techniques may not help them to remember tasks or events. Even though they remember past events, they often cannot relate the past to what is occurring now. People can live two to 20 years with Alzheimer's, although it commonly runs its course in about eight years. Even with good care and even in people with a strong constitution or will to live, Alzheimer's shortens a person's expected life span.

The risk of becoming afflicted with Alzheimer's increases with age, especially after age 75, and tends to run in families. Even so, except in rare cases, no one can predict who will become afflicted with Alzheimer's and when they will develop symptoms. Many people with Alzheimer's are the first in their families to be diagnosed with it.

In spite of similar losses, people with Alzheimer's are more different from each other than alike.

All Dementias Are Not AD

Alzheimer's is the most common—but not the only—cause of memory loss in middle-aged and older people. A common related disorder is Dementia with Lewy Bodies or Lewy Body Dementia (LBD), which basically is AD with Parkinson's symptoms. People with LBD have more problems with attention and concentration, and may have more falls and sudden confusional states during which they see or believe things that are not based in reality.

Vascular dementias such as Binswanger's disease and multi-infarct dementia are associated with small or large strokes and a history of high blood pressure, though many people with vascular dementia have Alzheimer's as well. Frontotemporal Lobe Dementia (FTD), or Pick's Disease, causes early changes in personality, lapses in judgment, and inappropriate behavior and is more common in younger people. There also are dementias associated with Parkinson's disease, chronic alcoholism, Huntington's disease, end-stage AIDS, and some rare rapidly progressive dementias like Creutzfeldt Jakob. People with Down's Syndrome, if they live long enough, are at high risk of developing a dementia.

Dementia occurs when a disease process damages thinking, perceiving, reasoning, language, and remembering. Dementia describes the symptoms; it is not a specific disease. A comprehensive medical evaluation is a must as soon as symptoms of dementia appear. Most of the time, a good medical evaluation will suggest a specific disease, course of treatment, and plan of care. A good medical evaluation includes laboratory, memory, and neurological tests and must include talking to someone who has known the person well over time.

There is no single blood test or X-ray that can identify AD. A qualified doctor must put together the results of all of the examinations, testing, and questioning to make a diagnosis. A brain autopsy after death remains the only sure way to confirm Alzheimer's.

What Happens To People With AD?

People with memory disorders lose functions, such as recent memory, reasoning, words, and a sense of time and place, at different rates, but most people with Alzheimer's have moments when they seem fine or when they can do things that they have not been able to do in quite some time. With the right kind of help and understanding, most people with Alzheimer's prefer to continue to be independent for as long as possible. But since the disease is progressive, people with Alzheimer's need more help over time. Just trying harder to remember or to perform tasks necessary for independent living does not work. It only frustrates people with Alzheimer's.

People with Alzheimer's know and remember that they are adults. They remember that they always took care of themselves. Because Alzheimer's develops slowly and often invisibly, it is hard to tell when it starts and even harder for many people to recognize that it is happening to them or to someone close to them. Some people with Alzheimer's are aware that something is different and may describe it as feeling "not right," lost, or in a fog. Others do not see themselves changing and resent being reminded that they are forgetting things. Families and facility staff may observe several changes during the first stages of Alzheimer's. These include:

- Memory loss that affects job skills;
- Difficulty performing familiar tasks;
- Problems with language;
- Disorientation to time and place;
- Poor or decreased judgment;
- Problems with abstract thinking;
- Misplacing things;
- Changes in mood or behavior;
- Changes in personality; and
- Loss of initiative.

Even when people exhibit obvious changes in memory, thinking, and naming things, they retain skills they have learned and practiced during a lifetime. Many people retain social skills and can make casual conversation or tell vivid or funny stories from the past. They may use these social skills to cover up mistakes or to make up explanations to fill in gaps in their memory. Other people can play the piano, sing songs they learned as children, or even play games they have known well. People with Alzheimer's want to continue to do things that remind them of their adult identities, skills, gifts, and special talents whenever possible. They will talk about work, their careers, their parents, or events from the distant past as if they happened yesterday.

On the other hand, people with Alzheimer's lose the ability to do many things that were part of their lives. As a result, they may feel useless and depressed or become frustrated and angry.

Although they may look fine, they are disabled. New learning and making new memories is hard, so they need guidance and reminders. People with Alzheimer's often forget that they forget. They are likely to forget a recent conversation, activity, or visit. They repeat themselves because they do not remember having asked or said the same thing already. Many people with Alzheimer's become worried, nervous, sad, or withdrawn. They may be afraid because their world does not make sense to them. They will, over time, have trouble paying attention to conversations or events, and they can be easily distracted.

People with Alzheimer's also lose the ability to recognize familiar objects and their use. They may try to wash clothes in the dishwasher or store refrigerator food in the pantry. They also may take other people's belongings and assume they are their own. Many people with Alzheimer's forget where they are or how to get where they want to go, even if their destination is only to the same dining room or bathroom they use many times each day. Even when they are in the bathroom, they may not remember what to do there. They also have trouble following cues or instructions, especially if there is more than one step. Having properly fitting prescription glasses and hearing aids at least makes sure that visual and auditory messages are received. People with Alzheimer's may be able to read a clock or a calendar date, but they may not know what the numbers mean. Thirty minutes may seem like 30 days to them, so saying, "I'll be back in a minute" has no meaning. They may forget names and start calling a daughter "that girl" or staff "those people."

Changes in behavior, personality, mood, and function are very common traits of Alzheimer's disease. Some personality traits, such as excessive worrying or suspiciousness, can become more extreme with Alzheimer's. People with Alzheimer's sometimes experience personality changes that upset family and friends. People who were trusting may become suspicious, and people who were thoughtful and agreeable may become withdrawn, irritable, or indifferent to others' feelings. Some people with Pick's Disease act silly or childlike. It's the disease that causes the childlike behavior—not the adult becoming a child.

Unfortunately, needing help does not make everyone receptive to receiving help. People with Alzheimer's may resent or resist help even when they need it. Some people become bossy and demanding while others do not ask for help even when they are in danger. After awhile, individuals with Alzheimer's forget public versus private behavior. They may undress in public or say inappropriate or insensitive things that they would not have said before the illness. People who never cursed may curse. People who were fancy dressers may want to wear the same mismatched clothing every day, even when it needs washing.

People with AD misplace, hide, and lose things and may accuse those around them of stealing. Others may believe that their husbands or wives are having an affair or mistake another resident or staff member for a spouse. Some people hear their mother calling to them or see children or "little people" who are not really there. They may mistake shadows for scary animals, or they may think their room is a jail or hotel room. If their last clear memory is of a job or of being a boss, the resident may wander outside the facility trying to get to work.

People with Alzheimer's may develop fears of running water or misunderstand the reason they are being asked to undress in front of a stranger such as a nurse assistant. They also may become mixed up and use shaving cream for toothpaste. Even when they are physically able to bathe themselves, they may get out of the tub right after climbing in. They may forget to eat, forget how to eat, or eat things that are not food. They may forget to drink and could become seriously dehydrated without constant surveillance by nursing staff.

Thinking and trying to keep everything straight tires people with Alzheimer's. They need frequent breaks or rest between periods of stimulation and socialization. Even people who formerly kept very busy may enjoy watching rather than participating in an activity. AD affects sleep, so residents with Alzheimer's may sleep all day and stay up at night, have trouble going to sleep or staying asleep, or they may want to sleep all the time. Many people with Alzheimer's wake from a dream and believe they are still in the dream. Similarly, many people with Alzheimer's think that scenes on television are happening to them. They also may believe that their reflection in the mirror is another person following them. Because they cannot remember what was just said or what is actually happening to them, they need repeated reassurance that they are safe and that everything is under control.

Does Alzheimer's Worsen Over Time?

Eventually, people with Alzheimer's need more help with routine tasks like dressing, bathing, eating, and using the bathroom. They may need to have their clothing laid out in the order it will be put on. Pull-on clothing, like jogging suits or sneakers with Velcro closures, is easier to put on than clothing with snaps, buttons, or zippers, and should be offered unless the resident resists using pull-on clothing because it does not fit with the resident's self image.

People with Alzheimer's lose the ability to use or understand words. Sometimes, they will say the opposite of what they mean or use a similar sounding word that has a different meaning than the one they want to use. Some people begin to use their native language, even if they have spoken English for the past 50 years. Therefore, people who care for Alzheimer's residents have to become detectives, taking clues from behavior, appearance, and mood to find out what the resident needs or wants. A person with Alzheimer's looking for a toilet may pull at his clothing or just become agitated. Later in the disease, people with Alzheimer's may experience pain they are unable to describe in words.

Instead, they may tug at a sore arm or scream when transferred from the bed to a chair. They may repeat phrases like "come here" or "help me" without being able to describe the pain or what would make them feel better.

Eventually, almost everyone who lives long enough with Alzheimer's also forgets how to walk, loses the ability to control bowels and bladder, and cannot eat or drink independently. Because of problems with choking, most people with Alzheimer's need thickened drinks or pureed foods, and it may take extra time and skill to feed someone with Alzheimer's. Due to incontinence and immobility, skin breakdown and frequent infections may speed the decline from Alzheimer's. People with Alzheimer's often die of repeated infections such as pneumonia.

Can People With Alzheimer's Suffer From Depression?

Depression is very common in people with Alzheimer's, although the signs may not be easily recognizable. People with Alzheimer's may deny being sad or depressed. However, when they become depressed, they take no pleasure in things they used to enjoy. They may withdraw from people and activities they once loved, refuse to join in activities, or repeat negative statements like "I'm no good to anyone." Often, the symptoms of depression are only disinterest or increased irritability, frustration, or mood swings. People with Alzheimer's and depression appear to have lost their spark or zest for life.

The good news is that antidepressant medicines often work well in treating people with Alzheimer's—improving their mood, energy, attention, and ability to follow what is going on around them. Nondrug treatments for depression make the medicine work even better. Many depressed people with Alzheimer's start to feel and look better with more one-to-one attention. They may need someone to help them focus on an activity they enjoy. It helps to validate residents' feelings by assuring them that they have a right to feel bad about their losses. Exercise can be therapeutic; on the other hand, pep talks or suggestions to "snap out of it" are not helpful. It is important to encourage socialization and friendships in residents with Alzheimer's without pushing them into friendships or situations in which they are uncomfortable or unhappy.

What About Sudden Increased Confusion In People With Alzheimer's?

People with Alzheimer's are at high risk of delirium, especially when they are hospitalized. Delirium is a medical emergency that often is mistaken for a worsening of Alzheimer's symptoms. Delirium usually is caused by a medical condition, such as an undiagnosed infection. It also may be caused by poor nutrition or multiple medications. Any sudden change in abilities, behavior, alertness, or confusion necessitates an immediate medical evaluation. Prompt treatment of the medical condition causing the delirium will help the person return to the previous level of functioning.

Can Alzheimer's Be Cured?

Alzheimer's can be treated but not cured. Some people with mild cognitive impairment are taking part in studies to see if the more obvious signs of Alzheimer's can be delayed or prevented with the use of certain medications. Medicines called cholinesterase inhibitors (like Aricept or Exelon) can improve memory, thinking, and attention in people with mild to moderate Alzheimer's disease.

Antidepressant medicines like Zoloft, Paxil, or Trazedone can improve mood and sleep and limit excessive worry when used appropriately. Antipsychotic medications such as Risperdal, Zyprexa, or Haldol, and even some antiseizure medicines, are used when people with Alzheimer's are very agitated or when they believe, hear, or see things that are not real but are scary. Antipsychotics also are used to calm people with Alzheimer's who hurt themselves or others, until nondrug approaches can be put in place.

Good medical and nursing care is essential for people with Alzheimer's disease, but it is only the beginning of what can be done to treat the disease and, more important, to treat the person with the disease.

Starting Points For Care

1. People with Alzheimer's are more different than alike. The best teacher is often experience with each resident over time. However, what works today may not work tomorrow.
2. Staff cannot cure Alzheimer's disease or teach residents with Alzheimer's to remember recent events. However, staff can help to improve the quality of residents' lives and the quality of their visits with family and friends.
3. Most residents with Alzheimer's are not deliberately stubborn or ungrateful. The brain damage generally makes them behave differently than they would if they had a choice. Their behavior is beyond rational explanation or willful control. However, residents with Alzheimer's are more positive if they are treated well and supported by safe, reassuring environments and caregivers.
4. People with Alzheimer's are doing the best they can. Over time, they will need more help with dressing, bathing, eating, and very basic activities. Alzheimer's is a degenerative and progressive disease that gets worse over time. If a resident resists care, a caregiver can try to distract the resident by talking about an upcoming meal or family visit while assisting with ADLs.
5. People with Alzheimer's need to feel they are giving as well as receiving. They need meaningful things to do. Most people with AD do not like to be reminded of what they can no longer do for themselves.
6. AD and related disorders require a person-centered approach to care. Person-centered care begins with talking to the person and not about him. It means giving the person a chance to do something with you rather than doing something to him. It recognizes the healing aspects of having fun, playing, and celebrating. It also means knowing how to simply be with someone who is upset. Person-centered care means trying to understand where the person is in time and

what gives meaning to her life. Expressive arts that use all the senses give people a chance to express themselves when words become more difficult to use. Person-centered care means quiet time alone or with others to unwind from the stress of trying to understand what is happening and what is expected. Finally, person-centered care is giving just enough supportive help to complete an activity successfully.

7. AD and related disorders require a family-centered approach to care. Most people do not develop this disease in isolation. They have a personal history and a network of relationships that must be preserved. Staying connected to family and friends or creating new friendships or family in a facility is critical to quality of life.

8. Activities help people with Alzheimer's feel normal and useful. That's why work-related activity, entertainment, and even self-care, like applying lipstick, are important to residents with Alzheimer's. Activity programming helps residents with Alzheimer's express themselves in ways that still work for them. Meaningful activities have a purpose—the resident understands why he is doing them. Meaningful activities are not forced (the resident can say "no") and respect the resident's age and experience. Successful activities take advantage of what the resident can still do, promise success, and make the resident feel good right away. A successful activity program is one that incorporates everyone—activity professionals, nursing staff, residents, families, housekeepers, dietary staff, and groundskeepers. To personalize activities, find out past life experiences of residents. For example, ask about a resident's career, education, military experience, family history, achievements, losses, traumas, hobbies, tastes, likes and dislikes, personality, fears, sources of pride, and preoccupations.

A DAY IN THE LIFE OF MISS ABIGAIL

The following scenario presents an ideal person-centered day in the life of a resident with AD.

Jane, the nurse assistant, sees Miss Abigail beginning to waken. Jane opens the curtains, takes Miss Abigail's hand, and says, "Good morning, Miss Abigail. It looks like you and I are up with the birds." Jane makes casual conversation about the morning routine before asking Miss Abigail if she is hungry. Miss Abigail has trouble waking up and thinks she is in a dream. The mention of food motivates her to waken fully and accept bathroom assistance. Jane offers to help her "get started," reminding Miss Abigail that everybody can use a little help in the morning. Jane talks about the breakfast menu while she assists Miss Abigail with the toilet, washing up, and taking her medication.

Jane gives her the choice of wearing a robe or her jogging suit to breakfast. She takes Miss Abigail's hand and they walk together toward Miss Abigail's table in the small dining room, wondering out loud whether her friend and dining partner, Miss Bethany, will be there before her. Miss Bethany is seated and Miss Abigail is offered decaffeinated coffee as she sits with her companion. The dining room staff take over, offering the ladies one item of food at a time, allowing time between items to encourage conversation between the two residents. When they are finished, the dining staff suggest that the women continue their conversation while sitting outside, where they will have a better view of Miss Abigail's bird feeder.

On the patio, an activity staff member is starting to water the raised plant beds and refill the bird feeders. She asks Miss Abigail for help, then asks if she and her friend would please help in the activity room. On the way to the activity room, they pass the bathroom and decide to stop there first. The friends then are asked to select the music for morning exercises. Chair exercise to music is followed by some ball toss. Next, Miss Abigail is asked if she has time to help wipe the tables before crafts begin. During this period, one resident is playing the piano, others are wiping tables, and still others are sweeping the floor. A few men are stacking chairs in the corner. Staff thank each resident for their contribution and suggest that everyone might need a break. Miss Abigail is given her favorite magazine and seated in a comfortable chair by the window. Later, there is a 20-minute arts program before Miss Abigail returns to her room for private time before lunchtime entertainment.

Each day before lunch a staff member, family visitor, or resident provides a special presentation. The same program may be repeated frequently. Staff with musical talent may sing or play an instrument, a resident may tell a funny story, or Miss Abigail may report about the kinds of birds visiting her feeder. Residents are encouraged to socialize with each other and guests before going to the dining room for the main meal of the day. Miss Abigail and Miss Bethany have a table to themselves because they are most comfortable eating together. They may share food because they are on similar diets. Today, Miss Abigail's nephew joins them for lunch. He thanks them for including him.

After lunch, the ladies "retire" to their rooms to rest after a busy morning. Miss Abigail prefers to rest in her recliner with her favorite throw over her legs. Later in the afternoon, Miss Abigail is invited to tea in the parlor, which is accompanied by conversation about china patterns and favorite serving pieces. Afternoon tea is hosted by different facility volunteers and family visitors each day to free up staff for shift change and report. A few men may wander in to the tea party but they generally return to the men's group watching sports or safari videos in the activity room. After tea, Miss Abigail will return to her room to arrange her animal collection on her shelves, watch a favorite show, and use the bathroom before supper.

After supper, residents are encouraged to relax in the living room where card games, checkers, and puzzles are left out on tables. Tonight, Miss Abigail's former neighbor stops by to visit in Miss Abigail's room. When her visitor leaves, a nurse assistant brings Miss Abigail her terry bathrobe and offers her a warm bath to help her sleep. Through trial and error, the staff has discovered that she is more comfortable bathing in the evening than in the morning. Once in the tub, she is offered a soapy washcloth and help with her shampoo. When she returns to her room, the assistant always asks Miss Abigail's preferences about room lighting, blankets, and temperature before wishing her sweet dreams and reminding her that she will be close by if she needs anything. Before leaving, the assistant hands Miss Abigail a soft pillow she cross-stitched as a child.

What Makes This A Person-Centered Approach To Care?

1. Staff personalize Miss Abigail's wake-up ritual with things she enjoys, such as a quiet breakfast with a resident she likes, talk about her bird feeder, and a visit outside to enjoy the morning.
2. Activities that interest and comfort Miss Abigail are offered throughout the day, such as guiding her to her favorite chair with a favorite magazine to rest, offering companionship during the day, and encouraging her nephew to visit with Miss Abigail and her companion at mealtimes.
3. Staff acknowledge special needs and comfort objects, such as Miss Abigail's favorite throw, cross-stitch pillow, and terry robe.
4. Miss Abigail is offered a choice whenever possible, including with clothing, food items, and activities.

Chapter

RESPONDING TO CHALLENGING BEHAVIORS

The following scenes take a close look at specific behaviors that may exist with AD. Each behavioral symptom or group of symptoms is illustrated with a story. Each story is then followed with a description of how and why the behavior might happen and ways to limit or prevent its reoccurrence. Helping strategies are listed under the following headings:

- Communicating With The Resident;
- Activities Of Daily Living;
- Activities; and
- Environmental Strategies.

Each category includes tips for talking to the resident; adapting personal care assistance to prevent the behavior in the future; using activities, arts, and music to prevent the behavior; and adapting the surroundings to match the resident's needs. At the end of each scenario, a three-point tip checklist is provided for quick review.

These suggestions are just a beginning. Try one or two and see how they work. Try others until you find solutions you are comfortable using. Add your ideas to each story. If these suggestions do not fit your style or facility, try others. Brainstorming with other staff and residents' families will help you tailor approaches. Creativity and flexibility are the keys to successful AD care. Your creativity and "tricks of the trade" will grow as you experiment with what works.

It is not necessary to memorize a list of solutions for each possible behavioral challenge. Remembering the process for helping to diffuse a challenging moment—trying to find out what's going on, communicating with the resident, and altering the environment—is the most important step toward effective caregiving. Remember: staff, family, and visitors must do the changing and responding. Residents with Alzheimer's cannot understand the need for change nor how to accomplish it.

Changes In Behavior

People with Alzheimer's generally are not intentionally difficult, irrational, stubborn, or angry. They simply cannot explain their needs or frustrations as they once could. Sometimes Alzheimer residents become angry when they feel out of control or when they are asked to do more than they can handle. Assume that residents with Alzheimer's are distressed by their loss of control and independence. They need help, support, and guidance. Residents with Alzheimer's are adults and must be treated with dignity and respect at all times. Treating adults like children only makes things worse for everyone, especially Alzheimer residents, who are very sensitive to tone of voice and body language. They can "read" your gritted teeth, anger, impatience, rolling of your eyes, or shaking your head or a finger at them. Residents with Alzheimer's are more cooperative and trusting when they feel competent, successful, and understood.

A Framework For Compassionate Caregiving

As people with Alzheimer's become more unsure of their surroundings or of what's expected of them, they become more dependent on staff, family, and often, other residents. As they lose the ability to understand their surroundings and our expectations, many people with Alzheimer's fear being left alone or forgotten. Therefore, when working with AD residents, follow these steps:

- Walk toward the resident slowly from the front, moving to the side, crouching at head-to-head level, and letting the resident know you are coming by making eye contact or offering the resident your hand.
- Identify yourself and call the resident by a name that she likes to be called. Do not ask if the resident remembers you.
- Take time for pleasantries before easing into tasks.
- Speak slowly, in a low pitch, and direct your words to the person's good ear.
- Use familiar words and short ideas but watch the tone of your voice—do not speak with disrespect.
- A gentle touch, nod, or smile offers confidence to a frightened resident.
- Offer guided choices between two acceptable options.
- Watch for signs of restlessness or withdrawal. Try again later if necessary.
- Ask one question at a time and wait for a response. Respond to the feeling behind the words.
- Use statements like "let's go" rather than "Are you ready to go now?" People with Alzheimer's often say "no" when asked if they would like to do something.
- Say "come with me" and avoid slang like "jump in."
- Use cues like pointing, touching, smiling, demonstrating, or starting the motion.
- Reduce confusing background noise or activity during a conversation.
- Be calm, open, adult, and positive.
- If you do not understand a resident's comment, ask her to show you or let you try again.
- Help to find a missing word by guessing and asking if you are on the right track.
- Ask questions that can be answered with a "yes" or "no."
- Say "good," "yes," "that's it" along the way when things are going well. People who live in the moment need praise and reassurance in the moment as well.
- Keep promises. If you forget something, admit it. Residents will be more comfortable if you admit mistakes.
- Be gracious in exiting. Say, "It was good to see you. You take care."

The Ten Absolutes

Never ARGUE instead AGREE
Never REASON instead DIVERT
Never SHAME instead DISTRACT
Never LECTURE instead REASSURE
Never say REMEMBER instead REMINISCE
Never say I TOLD YOU instead REPEAT
Never say YOU CAN'T instead say DO WHAT YOU CAN
Never COMMAND or DEMAND instead ASK or MODEL
Never CONDESCEND instead ENCOURAGE and PRAISE
Never FORCE instead REINFORCE

—*Jo Huey, from her book "Alzheimer's Disease: Help and Hope." Reprinted with permission.*

Unraveling Challenging Behaviors

- Remember: Behavior has meaning and can be a symptom of the illness or a response to a stressful environment.
- Rethink: Is the behavior harmful or scary to the resident or others, or can you accept it?
- Redirect: If a resident is pacing, agitated, or scared, provide a more positive activity, such as a walk, a dusting job, or a memory box to sort through.
- Remind: Take every chance to greet and let the resident know that you think of her often.
- Restrict: Stop the person from doing things that are harmful. Take dangerous objects from the room.
- Celebrate and capitalize on retained skills. Give a former nurse a clipboard for charting, for example.
- Create moments of fun.
- Distract: Snacks, treats, a cup of tea, a rock in the rocker, an offer of a manicure, or even a hug may divert or calm an agitated resident.
- Soothe: Note security objects that reassure and comfort a resident—a sweater over the shoulder or a favorite hat or

purse can be offered when the resident is upset.
- Reassure: Say, "I know you're upset. May I help you?" If a resident is searching frantically, calmly join in her search while suggesting that you know you can find the lost item together. Let her know she is not alone and that you understand how important the missing item is to her.
- Be present: Nothing comforts better than standing by a resident who is upset, offering sympathy, understanding, a shoulder to cry on, a tissue, or a knowing kind look. Do not ask a lot of questions.
- Routines, rituals, repetition: Knowing what will happen next reassures people with Alzheimer's. Bedtime or late afternoon rituals help, such as handing a resident her favorite afghan or playing her favorite audiotape or videotape.
- Slow down and simplify: Avoid busy, crowded, or noisy places when the resident is upset or needs to concentrate on a task. Rushing scares and confuses people with Alzheimer's.
- Back down from accomplishing tasks if the resident becomes upset. Say, "This isn't a good time for us to do this. Let's try again later."
- Break down big tasks into small pieces: Provide one-step guidance and tell the resident that you two are doing fine after each step.
- Compensate: Do for her what she can no longer do with ease.
- Let forgetting work for the resident. Don't remind, argue, scold, lecture, or confront a resident after an outburst.
- Safety precautions help: Prevent wandering or accidents by disguising exits with stop signs or black floor mats, or by alarming exits.
- Register residents with the Safe Return program through the Alzheimer's Association. Safe Return is a national program to help identify people who wander and become lost. Registered individuals receive a bracelet and clothing labels with a toll-free crisis number, and alert others that the individual is memory impaired and may need assistance.
- Be a model: Let other caregivers see you reassure or distract a resident so they can learn from your approach.

OFF AND RUNNING

"How do I get to Martin County from here?"

Mr. Pearce is an 82-year-old African American man with Alzheimer's living in a rural North Carolina residential care facility. He is always on the move. In fact, staff have learned to dress him while he walks. He mumbles constantly, "Gotta get there, fixin' to go there," and asks repeatedly how far it is to the Martin County line, site of his childhood home. He walks in circles through the facility and actually wears out the soles of his shoes. He has a history of wandering at night, and over time the local sheriff has learned where he is headed and finds him quickly. His social worker wants him transferred to a secured skilled facility, but the closest available bed is 200 miles from his daughter, who does not want him living so far from her.

What's Going On?

Anyone with Alzheimer's is at risk of wandering. People who wander away unnoticed from long term care facilities are described as "eloping." Dozens of possible reasons can be behind Mr. Pearce's need to wander. Consider some of the following:

- Medications—These may cause increased restlessness or confusion and lead to wandering.
- Stress—Is there too much noise or confusion in the environment? Is Mr. Pearce being asked to do more than he thinks he can do? Is he worried that someone is waiting for him?
- Time confusion—Sometimes people wake from a dream at night and without any light or familiar things around them, believe they are somewhere in their dream. Mr. Pearce may think he's back 50 years ago when his job required him to return to Martin County by a certain time each night.
- Basic needs—Mr. Pearce may be searching for food, a drink,

or the outhouse of his childhood.

- Visuospatial problems—Mr. Pearce may want to sit, but cannot remember how to position his body in a chair, so he keeps on moving.
- Restlessness—Maybe Mr. Pearce needs more structured activity and exercise for stimulation and is pacing because he does not know what to do.
- Unfamiliarity—Mr. Pearce may be searching for a place, person, or job.
- Fear—Does Mr. Pearce feel threatened by someone in the facility? Perhaps another resident reminds him of a supervisor who was critical of him.
- Old routine—Was Mr. Pearce a man who worked nights or was he always a worrier who walked the floor at night when he couldn't sleep?

By learning about Mr. Pearce—his habits, history, preferences—staff may be able to discover reasons for his wandering and can then adapt the environment or schedule to fulfill his needs.

Strategies That Work

Communicating With Mr. Pearce

Staff can walk with Mr. Pearce while they are talking. He may be more comfortable with this side-by-side style of conversation. Check to see if he is looking for food, a bathroom, a drink, or if he is feeling lost. To guide him back inside when he wanders out of the facility, tell him it is a long way to the county line, and you are sure he will want his hat or a drink before he goes. Once inside, engage in a discussion of which hat or beverage he would prefer and let forgetting work for him.

Ask him to tell you about Martin County—what does he do there? Talk with other staff and figure out if there is a way to incorporate his old job routines into the routine at the facility.

Since his daughter, Gloria, visits regularly, remind Mr. Pearce that she will be looking for him here. Ask him to stay around just until his daughter arrives. In the meantime, ask him to help you carry or move something. He is probably strong enough to move or stack empty boxes or chairs. Perhaps he could deliver newspapers or fliers to each person's room to encourage conversation and breaks along his way.

Make sure—prior to admission—that Mr. Pearce's daughter understands that there is no fail-safe method to keep people with Alzheimer's from wandering. Tell her what your facility can do to prevent further episodes of night wandering beyond becoming a secured or locked dementia care facility. Ask her which strategies are acceptable to her. Would she be willing to contribute to a wandering tracking device for him? Also, invite Gloria to a care planning meeting and develop a detailed plan for keeping Mr. Pearce occupied and within sight of staff. If Mr. Pearce is most likely to try to leave in the late afternoon, maybe Gloria or a volunteer could visit at that time for a walk. Everyone should be clear about procedures if he does exit unnoticed. A time should be set to review the plan and discuss possible changes. Staff should make every effort to support Gloria's preference to keep her father at this facility while acknowledging the risks. It should be made clear that this is a quality of life issue for him and that it may mean taking risks.

In addition, ask her for suggestions for activities that would interest and engage her father, and see if she knows why her father is focused on returning to the Martin County line. Is there a specific phrase that can be used to reassure him that he is living up to expectations?

Activities Of Daily Living

Mr. Pearce forgets and walks away in the middle of personal care and dressing. He needs someone to show him what to do one step at a time and, sometimes, start it for him.

1. Make sure Mr. Pearce has clothing that can be put on easily, such as pants with an elastic waistband and pullover shirts. He needs sturdy supportive shoes with Velcro closures and special attention to foot care.
2. Perhaps Mr. Pearce would be more cooperative with a male assistant. His daughter jokes that he was "quite the ladies' man." A male assistant could offer him privacy and remind him that there are ladies out there, and he will want to look nice when he leaves the room.
3. Make personal care fun and special. Offer him a nice after-shave after shaving and have him admire how nice he looks when groomed.
4. Mr. Pearce has difficulty getting in a bathtub, so try a shower. Talk him through a shower with stories of his boyhood in Martin County. Mr. Pearce also may like singing in the shower.
5. If he does leave his room without his shirt, start walking with him and casually mention that you "noticed" he is looking for his shirt and you have it. Sometimes you might have to finish dressing him in the hall.
6. Mr. Pearce is likely to get up and leave a meal before it is served. Some facilities use rituals like saying grace or singing show tunes to remind people to stay seated until the meal is served. Give him something to drink immediately after he sits and ask him if he will keep his dining partners company while you bring in the rest of the meal. Some people indicate their restlessness by asking to be excused. They may need a smaller dining table or less stimulation. Mr. Pearce may need finger foods that he can eat while walking around the facility.

Activities

Mr. Pearce needs vigorous activity throughout the day and evening, with frequent breaks or catnaps in a rocker, glider, or other chair that is easy for him to get in and out of. Outdoor structured work activities would be an ideal choice: gardening, stacking wood, digging, raking, or even rearranging porch chairs may be engaging and help him feel productive. One clever staff person kept a man engaged in stacking wood far beyond his usual attention span. She kept thanking him, asking him if it was time for him to go "on break," joking with him about how watching him work made *her* tired, and suggesting that he send her the bill.

Invite Mr. Pearce to join all music and singing activities by letting him know that you need his strong voice to round out the group. He might be just the resident to engage in spontaneous dancing when the music is on, whether in the activity room or even in the hall or dining room before dinner. Finally, Mr. Pearce might enjoy a box of his favorite and most interesting items to sort through or look at when he does take a break.

Environmental Strategies

Always be prepared—any person with Alzheimer's may leave at any time. But do not assume that the resident wants to leave you or the facility. He may only be searching for something.

Steps to discourage wandering into unfamiliar areas or leaving the facility include:

- At night, a pressure-sensitive mat at the door to his room may alert staff when Mr. Pearce is out of his room. A door alarm system or a tracking device that sounds an alarm when Mr. Pearce leaves a defined area can be considered as well. Disguising or changing exits wanderers normally use, such as installing screens or displaying stop signs in front of doors, is another subtle change that may prevent wandering.

- At a minimum, Mr. Pearce should wear a nonremovable identification bracelet at all times.
- Mr. Pearce's room may need more "Martin County" reminders so he will feel more at home. His daughter can bring items he finds reassuring, or staff can hang a sign on the wall of his room, away from the door, that says "Martin County Line."
- Mr. Pearce's room should be visible from a staff area for constant surveillance.
- Walking in circles is not interesting. Create a more interesting path for Mr. Pearce through the facility. Consider enclosing an outdoor area with activities that draw him and others outside without having to go in small circles. At a minimum, create a winding path through a safe area of the facility for him to use.
- Use awnings or other attractive entrances to rooms that Mr. Pearce should explore, such as into the dining room or activity areas.
- Involve local law enforcement—suggest that local law enforcement officers take training or review materials from the Alzheimer's Association about how to respond to people with Alzheimer's. Give them a current picture of Mr. Pearce, the name he responds to, and where he might tell an officer he is headed. Keep an article of his clothing with his scent on it in a freezer bag along with an imprint of the sole of his favorite shoe on aluminum foil. These items are helpful for tracking with dogs.
- Register him with the Alzheimer Association's Safe Return program.

Tip Checklist

1. Register residents who "elope" from the facility with Safe Return.
2. Consider a glider or rocking chair for restless residents.
3. Start walking with a resident who is leaving the facility and gradually guide the resident back inside.

RUMMAGING

"I know it's here and it's mine"

Miss Murphy is a 78-year-old, never-married, retired elementary school teacher who uses a wheelchair. She was diagnosed with Alzheimer's after her admission to the skilled nursing facility for physical therapy. She makes the rounds of other residents' rooms, rearranging their drawers, searching through and picking up other people's underwear, and stashing others' belongings in her chair or hiding them in her room. She says, "I know it's here someplace," as she moves in and out of rooms. She never takes things she needs— she usually has the same items in her room. She even takes food from the dining room after each meal. She acts insulted when she is told that the items taken do not belong to her or that this is not her room. She insists that she is not "that kind of person."

What's Going On?

Hiding things, hoarding unimportant items, taking others' belongings, and losing and searching for things are common symptoms of people with memory loss. People want to hang on to what is theirs to feel like themselves, but they cannot determine what belongs to them because nothing looks familiar. In addition, people with Alzheimer's have no idea where their next meal is coming from and it seems reasonable to them to put away some food "just in case." Because they lose recent memory, they cannot remember where things are hidden. They also forget where things go so they may put stale food in a dresser or a hearing aid in the wastebasket.

Tips For Rummagers

- All personal items should be marked with the owner's name.
- Label drawers or tape up pictures of which items go where in Miss Murphy's room.

- Have extras of things she seeks (like tissues) available when she starts looking.
- Set aside a drawer in her room with interesting items. Suggest that the drawer may contain the item she is looking for.
- Learn her favorite hiding places and always check wastebaskets before emptying them.
- Latch one drawer or closet in Miss Murphy's room where valuable items can be kept safe from rummaging.
- Stale food routinely should be removed from Miss Murphy's room and replaced with fresh snacks.
- Encourage staff, other residents, and families to keep a tolerant sense of humor about inevitable mix-ups of belongings.

Strategies That Work

Communicating With Miss Murphy

Miss Murphy may be hungry or looking for a bathroom, so staff should start walking with her and offer a snack or a chance to use the bathroom. Miss Murphy may be asked to accompany staff while checking in on other residents. It is easier to intercept or prevent incidents if Miss Murphy is in sight.

If staff see her leaving another resident's room with something that is not hers, staff should try to intercept the item by asking her to hold another object while taking the object she is holding. The item can be replaced later. If she takes a pillow from another resident's chair, staff could tell her that she does not look as comfortable with that one as she does with her favorite pillow, and replace her own pillow. When she is found in another resident's room, suggest that she cannot keep an eye on her favorite outdoor or indoor area from that room and that it is time for the two of you to check on her fish or birdfeeder. Find every opportunity to compliment her good taste and career achievements. Ask her to tell you about items in her room as a way of drawing her back to her room.

Activities Of Daily Living

1. Incorporate a discussion of "her things" into dressing and grooming. Talk about her special hairbrush and her lovely hand mirror, and point to the stack of fresh tissues on her dressing table.
2. After dining room meals, Miss Murphy can be encouraged to help collect napkins or some easily reachable items from the tables.
3. When helping Miss Murphy in and out of the wheelchair, offer to make some room for her by removing the items she has collected that day. Make sure she has a side bag that she can reach on her wheelchair that has her favorite security objects.

Activities

- Miss Murphy needs fresh air and exercise for mood, appetite, vitamins, and to promote sleep. Make sure scheduled and impromptu exercise is available indoors and outside.
- Miss Murphy tells everyone she is a retired teacher. Perhaps she would enjoy helping a staff member's child by "checking over his homework." Stacks of old school papers or books of children's writing can be kept in a desk in Miss Murphy's room for her to work on.
- Miss Murphy can be asked to help someone sort items for a school fundraiser.
- Sorting tasks or a sorting box of school supplies may engage her between small group activities. Be sure to thank her for her work, and resupply the box with different items if she loses interest.
- Miss Murphy could be invited to help lead upper-body exercise groups.
- Perhaps Miss Murphy could be given a stack of old school textbooks to evaluate.

- Miss Murphy needs a friend, such as another resident with similar interests or background or a volunteer who respects teachers.
- Be sure Miss Murphy is invited and escorted to all intergenerational programs or visits from school groups. Engage her in conversations about how schools and children's lives have changed since she started teaching school. Miss Murphy may be a good candidate for a special volunteer or "adopted" family.
- Encourage Miss Murphy to display collections in her room that she can rearrange daily.
- Use every chance to tell her that no one has anything like what she has in her room.

Environmental Strategies

- Warm, varied textures or familiar objects from long ago may meet some of Miss Murphy's searching needs. Let her have these objects in her room or in neutral territory like a small sitting room or activity area.
- Display certificates and awards that Miss Murphy received during her long teaching career. Photographs of her former students may offer pleasant opportunities for reminiscing.
- Miss Murphy needs a reason to go to an activity or public area. If there are interesting things accessible in public areas, she is less likely to go to other people's rooms in search of "her" things.
- If she regularly enters only certain private rooms, these doors should be kept shut, potentially with a "Do Not Disturb" or "Danger" sign that may be applied quickly at her eye level as she approaches.
- Fresh snacks, such as boxes of raisins or cereal bars marked with her name, can be left by her bed to reassure her that food is always available.

Tip Checklist

1. Discretely replace items that a resident "collects" from others without confronting the resident.
2. Lock valuables in one drawer. Set up a rummaging drawer for exploring in the resident's room.
3. Check for and remove stale food from resident rooms. Replace these items with fresh, healthy snacks that are easily visible.

AGGRESSION AND UNSAFE BEHAVIORS

"It came out of nowhere"

Dr. Piney is an 85-year-old retired surgeon living in the Alzheimer's unit of a skilled nursing facility. He is a friendly, dignified man whose wife encourages staff to call him "Doc" and to let him wear his old starched lab coats, which she launders and supplies in quantity. Dr. Piney has had a private-duty male assistant, Tony, ever since he climbed out a window and ate a bar of fancy soap that he mistook for a piece of chocolate. Dr. Piney likes Tony, but repetitively lectures to him as if he were a medical student.

When Tony arrived this morning, Dr. Piney was irritable and refused to get out of bed. Tony decided to offer him a wash-up in bed. He wrung out a washcloth and as he turned to start care, Dr. Piney grabbed Tony's wrist and started to bite his arm. Tony is much taller and much stronger than Dr. Piney, but he could not loosen the doctor's steel grip on his wrist. During the episode, Dr. Piney said, in an unusually indifferent way, "I gotta kill you." Dr. Piney has never been combative, aggressive, or even angry with Tony.

What's Going On?

It is virtually impossible to predict the timing and all the possible dangerous or unsafe behaviors of someone with dementia, because each resident perceives safety and threat differently. Even in the most secure environments, unprovoked combative or unsafe behavior may occur without warning and may seem to come out of nowhere. Sometimes it occurs only once, but often, if triggers for the behavior are not identified, the behavior will continue or get worse. Triggers to aggressive or agitated behaviors can be physical, like a new illness, pain, constipation, or impaction; environmental, like noisy or confusing environments; emotional, such as feeling that staff are tense or rushed; or not based in reality, such as when the resident's perceptions or responses to ideas inside his head cause him to act out.

The most common triggers for combative behavior are fear resulting from feelings of intrusion into one's personal space; misunderstanding or misperceiving a threat that isn't there; an inability to describe in words what is needed; or distress, depression, worry, or frustration.

Dr. Piney may have slept poorly, woken from a frightening dream, or not recognized Tony or his surroundings. It is possible that similar outbursts occurred at home, but his wife may have hesitated to report them on admission. She may have recognized his need for close supervision when she chose to employ Tony.

Strategies That Work

Preventing Aggressive Or Unsafe Behaviors

1. Be alert. Tony should proceed more slowly in the future. If Dr. Piney appears confused or upset, a gentle and careful approach is needed.
2. Have tabletop supplies available, such as Dr. Piney's stethoscope and a pocket-sized book of medication dosages, to reassure Dr. Piney. Tony could ask him to sign an admitting note or a prescription—a normalizing and distracting activity.
3. Ask for his help—do not tell him you are taking over.
4. Offer him a snack or treat.
5. Have a code to call for extra staff assistance if necessary. Sometimes, another person coming in and replacing Tony

will help Dr. Piney feel rescued from whatever threat he thought Tony posed.

6. Remove dangerous items from his room like razors, poisons, or confusing items like odd-shaped soaps.

7. Learn his nonverbal signs of increasing agitation: becoming red in the face, clenching his fists, rapidly searching with his eyes, or waving his hands in the air.

8. Learn his verbal signs of escalating anger—cursing, using a loud voice, or muttering.

9. Change the environment. If he is in the hallway, bring him to his room. If he is in bed, dim the lights and remind him that he put himself on bed rest until his illness cleared.

10. Reduce staff expectations of his performance and agree that it is okay to accomplish less in more time.

11. Slow down as the aggressive resident speeds up. Staff's nonverbal and verbal slowing can have a calming effect.

12. Never surround or gang up on an aggressive resident or someone who is about to attack, jump, or run. It can prompt a fight-or-flee response if the resident feels cornered or overwhelmed.

13. Tell him that staff will call one of his doctor friends for a consult since he does not look well. He may, in fact, have a change in his medical condition or response to medications that should be evaluated.

14. Dr. Piney may respond with aggression to medications for depression, anxiety, or pain.

15. Do not make any assumptions about what is safe. If Dr. Piney climbed out a window and ate soap, he may just as likely eat pennies out of a wishing well fountain as throw them in. He is also a risk to vulnerable or frail residents whom he may try to help—with potentially dangerous consequences.

Communicating With Dr. Piney

Talk in a soothing, calm tone of voice, and keep your comments simple. Try whispering in his ear, "Doc, can you look at my leg? I need a second opinion," or "I hear you, Doc, and I'll take care of it." If Dr. Piney starts to bite, staff should say, "let go," or "stop." If that does not stop the behavior, tell Dr. Piney, "You have a stat call," and offer him the telephone. Comfort Dr. Piney after the incident is defused. He will need reassurance that everything is under control. Suggest taking a deep breath together.

In response to his comment, "I gotta kill you," say "Let's get something for your pain now," or "Let's get a snack now," in a calm, quiet voice. While talking, press just above his wrist and use your weight to push his arm in close to his body. If he grabs your hair, squeeze his hand and move your head closer to his. Do not pull away.

Activities Of Daily Living

1. Delay personal care when Dr. Piney is upset. Suggest that he has had a hard night on-call and needs more sleep.
2. Suggest that he needs to wash up before going on rounds and that you are here to assist.
3. Give him gum to chew if he can chew and remember to spit it out safely. Residents who put things in their mouths or bite may need safe objects for sucking or chewing.
4. Have pillows around during bed care to protect Dr. Piney and you from punching, kicking, or grabbing. Hand him a pillow or towels to grab onto.
5. Move to the side or out of his direct vision but stay on his level when helping with bathing or personal care. He is less likely to feel attacked if the caregiver stays low and nonconfrontational.
6. He may need real physical reassurance, so staff should hold

him close and remind him that staff are here to protect him and keep him safe.

7. Keep his favorite treats or hard candy in his lab coat pocket or close by. Remind him that he needs a quick energy boost.

8. If he grabs your arm or wrist, stroke the lower arm of the grabbing hand or place your hand over his grabbing hand and squeeze firmly. As a last resort, move your finger under the jaw in front of the ear and push in and up.

9. If threatened with an object like a cane or chair, grab a safe object like a pillow that can stop the threatening object without causing harm. If a resident is physically threatening and abusive, the facility needs a medical consult to control the behavior. This is essential to protect other residents and staff.

10. Dr. Piney may need smaller dining groups, restaurant-style food, tablecloths, flowers, low lighting, and less noise at mealtimes. Give him space, one food at a time, and do not help more than he needs.

11. Offer a shampoo and shave in a barbershop atmosphere rather than one-on-one in a bathroom.

Activities

Leave old-fashioned medical charts and textbooks in Dr. Piney's room for review when he seems upset. To further incorporate his past life into the present, offer to accompany him on his rounds and engage him in conversation while he is walking around the facility. If he seems upset or eager to examine another resident, suggest that you go in a private area or outside to discuss the case first.

Find a small audience for Dr. Piney's repetitive lectures. Have them sit and have him stand or pace as preferred while he talks. Prompt him to say more. In addition, ask him to demonstrate exercises in a group exercise program or ask him if he thinks a particular exercise is good for the heart or the muscles.

Ask Dr. Piney what he enjoys most in his free time, and take advantage of his spontaneous selection of individual activities to build an activity plan around them. Perhaps he loved fishing, fine dining, or woodworking. Also, Dr. Piney may do well in a guided reminiscence group talking about career challenges, teaching, or even the stresses of raising children and having a busy career.

Find a "colleague" or special friend for Dr. Piney within the facility—it might be another resident from the same neighborhood, church, or profession. Friendships are reassuring because they can build new connections rather than focusing on lost ties. Some agitated residents respond best to "doctor's orders for bed rest." It absolves them of responsibility for more than they can handle at the time.

Environmental Strategies

A safe environment is essential for Dr. Piney. All dangerous objects should be removed from resident rooms. Personalize Dr. Piney's room with notes he can reread from grateful patients or pictures of special moments in his life like graduations, his wedding, or military service. A box of work or family memorabilia that he can tinker with to prompt reminiscing also may be useful. If Dr. Piney was a fisherman, a pillow with a joke about "gone fishin' " may prompt his sense of humor or encourage him to tell a funny story about fishing when he needs to calm down.

Have something in his room that his wife can work on when she visits. Dr. Piney may feel uncomfortable having to entertain visitors. If he is used to seeing his wife crocheting, clipping coupons, or working on her correspondence, he will feel more secure if she engages in these activities during visits.

Tip Checklist

1. Staff should slow down and remain calm in response to aggression.
2. Learn phrases that reassure residents who become agitated or aggressive.
3. Some aggressive residents may need to spend more time in bed, where they feel safe.

BATHING THE RESISTIVE RESIDENT

"I'm the man"

Mr. Rowling, a 78-year-old former football coach who has Alzheimer's, was admitted to an intermediate care wing of a nursing facility when his wife became terminally ill with cancer and could no longer care for him at home. He is a large, strong man who lumbers around like a former athlete. He refuses to participate in activities because his "war injuries keep acting up." He asks to see his doctor dozens of times in a conversation. When it is time for a bath, Mr. Rowling says, "No way." He says he takes care of those things. Mr. Rowling sweats and has developed an odor. He needs a bath but the nurse assistants are afraid he will overpower them.

What's Going On?

Mr. Rowling's last memory is that he is "The Man"—someone who can take care of himself. He is trying hard to maintain his "macho" identity by using familiar old phrases—like stating that his war injuries are "acting up." He may be asking for a doctor repeatedly because he thinks he is in the hospital or because he needs to feel comforted about needing help.

Strategies That Work

Communicating With Mr. Rowling

After learning from Mrs. Rowling that her husband always bathed before a big game, staff can suggest a shower "before the big game starts." Call him "Coach" if he prefers and give him something to look forward to, like being ready for the kickoff of the football game. To distract him from his repeated requests to call the doctor, staff can talk with Mr. Rowling about sports or his old army buddies.

Activities Of Daily Living

1. Show Mr. Rowling the bathing facility before asking him to use it. Ask him about the shower rooms in the army or school gym and how this shower room compares. Try a bath first thing in the morning before he gets dressed so he has less to do. In addition, have the family bring in his favorite robe or personalize a large terry robe by writing "Coach" or applying a favorite team emblem on it.

2. When he is ready for a bath, make sure the bathing room is warm. A heat lamp can be used as a prop "for therapy" for his injuries. Soft lighting eliminates glare. Use men's products with familiar scents like an old aftershave lotion.

3. If Mr. Rowling is frightened by his image in the mirror, cover it or spray something on it to temporarily cloud the image. If he enjoys talking to his image in a mirror, bring one in.

4. Have one person—the most trusted or favorite staff member, ideally a man—provide help with bathing to promote privacy. If he will not cooperate after several attempts, offer a towel or bed bath until "he feels more comfortable." Such a resident may be more comfortable with just one assistant, so make sure Mr. Rowling's bathing assistant carries a beeper in case of emergency.

5. Finally, do not ignore his need for a doctor—offer to do something that his doctor suggested to relieve his pain before attempting a bath, or tell him his doctor "ordered a hot whirlpool" before his visit. Of course, if Mr. Rowling appears to be in pain, or if his behavior changes dramatically, call his doctor to make sure he is not ill or requiring medical treatment.

6. When bathing Mr. Rowling, consider using his favorite music tape and singing along with him. Speak in soft tones and reduce equipment noise or noise from other staff conversations. Distract him with talk about the game.

7. Take one step at a time and say, "You're looking great" after each successful task. Give him a washcloth to hold and offer him a choice: "Do you want to wash your legs or should I?" Tell him what you are going to do before you do it. Be sure to check water temperature for him.
8. Let him stay covered with a towel except the part of his body being washed.
9. Shampoo last with a no-rinse shampoo or offer him a washcloth to put over his face. If he resists, consider delaying shampoo until he can go to a barbershop.
10. Ask him if there is anything else you can do to make him more comfortable.
11. After the bath, lay out his clothes in the order they should be put on and hand him one item at a time. Athletic clothes like jogging suits may be easier to put on and more familiar.
12. In addition, Mr. Rowling may be resistive to brushing his teeth or not do a very good job. Make sure his teeth are brushed well once a day at his most cooperative time using a small toothbrush. If he wears dentures, make sure they fit, are clean, and used regularly.

Handling Repetitive Requests

In addition to his resistance to bathing, Mr. Rowling also asks for the doctor repeatedly, despite the fact that a medical evaluation has revealed no basis for Mr. Rowling's complaints of pain. The following suggestions can help staff redirect a resident's repetitive requests.

1. Give Mr. Rowling a sign or note for his room saying the doctor wants to see him "in a week."
2. Provide him with a tablet to write down questions or requests for his doctor. Periodically take the list and tell him you will be sure it gets to the doctor.
3. Offer several comfort strategies to reduce the pain and distract him—and be sure to say that these are doctor's orders. Some residents with AD relive old war traumas. As a result,

Mr. Rowling may genuinely feel pain or terror.
4. Ask him to show you where it hurts and apply a lotion or heating pad to it. Tell him staff will keep trying until he is satisfied.
5. Encourage him by telling him that this place can help him recover from his injuries. Use the war injuries theme to go from the pain to conversation about his pride in service to his country.
6. People who ask repetitive questions are usually worried or unsure. Find ways to routinely escort or orient him to routines until he is more comfortable.

Activities

To engage Mr. Rowling in activities, direct him to men's or veterans' group meetings or sporting activities. Tell him it is time for the men's group and that they need him there. Offer him a pillow to put under his injured knee during the activity. Invite a current coach, player, or retired military officer to talk with the men's group about how coaching or the military has changed. Brief the guest on Mr. Rowling's successful career. Show a video or use pictures or old magazines to prompt a reminiscing session about the war. Ask Mr. Rowling, as a veteran, to help with flag raising or lowering daily.

Another idea is to ask him to help host a pancake breakfast for a local football team, or find a resident's family member who is willing to take him to a sports game. Ask him to tell you which young players have potential.

Environmental Strategies

- Make sure his mementos, trophies, and other recognitions are displayed prominently.
- His surroundings should encourage exercise, and he should be dressed in exercise-related clothing.

- A special easy chair in his room will help him take breaks.
- Mr. Rowling could be asked to help staff select exercise or sports equipment for the facility.

Tip Checklist

1. Save bathing for the resident's most calm, cooperative time of day.
2. Offer extra privacy with towels in the bathtub.
3. Some residents are less resistive to activities if they are "prescribed" by a doctor.

DELUSIONS, HALLUCINATIONS, AND MISIDENTIFICATIONS

"They are here again and I can't get a minute's peace"

Mrs. Levy is a 72-year-old nursing facility resident who has been diagnosed with Lewy Body Dementia. Her children admitted her following the death of her husband. Mrs. Levy is bothered by "little people" who come to her room at night to party. They are dirty and leave bugs that crawl up and down her arms. She calls her husband "shameless" for running around on her. Mrs. Levy is convinced that the youngest of her three children, her daughter Faith, who never visits, "is the only person left on this Earth I can trust." Mrs. Levy calls her other daughter, Caroline, by the name of Sarah, Mrs. Levy's deceased older sister. Sarah and Mrs. Levy had a falling out about their mother's money and did not speak to each other for years before Sarah died. Now "Sarah" is once again stealing her money.

Mrs. Levy has fallen several times at night trying to escape the little people in her room. When her son, Ray, and Caroline come for a visit, she looks helplessly at the staff and says, "Are you going to let that fat guy and his lady friend rob me blind? You better call Faith; she's the only person left on Earth I can trust." It is difficult for her devoted children to hear their mother heap praise on their absent sister. They say Mrs. Levy was a wonderful mother who never played favorites and never complained. It is also hard for them to see her become so weak and unsteady. When they ask her to eat more, she says, "How can I eat when I have no money for food? I sit here all day and no one invites me to dinner." After such episodes, Ray often races to the administrator with threats to sue for "neglect." Mrs. Levy's delusions, hallucinations, suspiciousness, and favoritism, along with her children's guilt and sorrow, present several challenges to the staff.

What's Going On?

Delusions

Delusions are fixed false beliefs that are not changed by presenting the facts or an explanation. Mrs. Levy believes that her children are stealing and that her husband is having an affair. Suspiciousness and delusions are common in people with memory loss, because memory loss often makes people think something is wrong, but they cannot identify the problem. Mrs. Levy, for instance, does not remember her last meal, but she does remember that adults pay for or buy food. Mrs. Levy cannot figure out what happened to her money or her husband. To protect her self image, she finds it easier to believe that "the fat man and his girlfriend" must have taken her money. Since her husband is not present, she assumes that he is off with other women. What is really stolen is her control, her freedom, and her memory. Mrs. Levy's delusions are a problem because her accusations upset her children and because her lack of understanding frightens her.

Hallucinations

People who hallucinate see, hear, smell, or feel things that are not there. Visual hallucinations like seeing little people are common with Lewy Body Dementia. Mrs. Levy also feels bugs crawling on her arms, a less common symptom. Hallucinations, like delusions, are not harmful if they are not scary and do not cause further problems for the resident or others. However, Mrs. Levy is troubled by her hallucinations and falls when rushing to escape. The hallucinations are interrupting Mrs. Levy's sleep, increasing her risk of falls, and triggering her fears of dirt or harm from the imaginary crawling bugs.

Misidentifications

People with memory loss often cannot remember their children as adults and easily confuse them with their own brothers and sisters. Mrs. Levy may think of her daughter as a girl of about eight years old. People with dementia also may think a husband is a father or a son is a brother. They are likely to call people by familiar well-practiced names from childhood, like substituting a sister's name for a daughter's. Some residents will call a current spouse by a former spouse's name for the same reason.

Strategies That Work

To prevent delusions, hallucinations, and misidentifications, try the following:

1. Check Mrs. Levy's hearing, vision, and clothing for textures that can cause "creepy crawly" sensations. Maybe giving her lotion and telling her it is bug repellent will take the sensation away.
2. Make sure cataracts or macular degeneration are not causing shadows that look like little people at night. Make sure she uses eyeglasses, hearing aids, and other corrective devices if they help.
3. Always check out the reality of accusations before offering reassurance. Children have been known to steal money from Mom's purse, and her husband may have had an affair during their marriage.
4. Turn on a night light in her room. Also, clear a path in her room to reduce the risk of falling.
5. Allow her to keep small amounts of money in a purse for easy inspection.
6. Keep an extra set of things she thinks are regularly stolen.
7. Some suspicious residents become more so if asked about things they do not remember, or if asked to be in a photograph.

8. Teach staff and family members not to become angry when accused of stealing from or cheating her. Make sure everyone understands that Mrs. Levy is not angry at them but at her situation.

9. Encourage Mrs. Levy's son to join her at mealtimes. He can be reassured that she is eating regularly.

10. Teach her family about her diagnosis and reinforce the idea that the delusions are not personal attacks.

Communicating With Mrs. Levy

Mrs. Levy needs a lot of reassurance that her needs will be taken care of at the facility. Tell her that meals are covered and that she is paid up.

When she has a delusion or hallucination, reassure her that, given what she sees and believes, she has a right to be upset or scared. Offer to clear the little people out of her room and lock them up so she can get some rest. Invite her to have a cup of tea with a staff person until her room is quiet again. Tell her, "I'm sorry you have had so much trouble in your room. Would it help if I held your hand or rubbed your back until you feel better?" Offer to check her arms and put on lotion to keep the bugs away or do a thorough bug check of her room. Help her feel understood by paying attention to her feelings, not her behavior or delusions. Avoid denying, confronting, arguing, or explaining what really happened. Be sure to let the doctor know if she hallucinates. Sometimes, medication is needed to treat delusions and hallucinations that are really threatening. Ask her daughter Faith to call and reassure her mother that she will make sure the bugs and little people are taken care of.

Also, reassure her children that you will not think less of their father because of their mother's accusations. Also, if Mrs. Levy says nice things about her son and daughter when she recognizes them in a picture, let them know that she retains pleasant memories of them. They may be encouraged to reminisce with her about a more pleasant time by using old photographs or mementos that she will connect to them as children.

Finally, do not tell her that her husband is dead. Instead, redirect the conversation from his alleged womanizing to how attractive he was and how nice they look together in their pictures. Encourage the children to remind their mother that she always came first in their father's eyes.

Activities Of Daily Living

1. Mrs. Levy should be escorted to meals and reassured that she is paid up each time.
2. Offer her extra nighttime snacks like warm milk to help her relax and to prevent dehydration.
3. Mrs. Levy can get extra calories from food served at a morning coffee club or afternoon social. Nutrient-dense recipes can be prepared for nighttime snacks when she cannot sleep.
4. Maintaining Mrs. Levy's mobility with her increasing risk of falls is an issue. She may need something to hold onto when she walks from her bed to the nurses' station.
5. Mrs. Levy may need to stay up with staff at night and sleep later in the morning.

Activities

- Mrs. Levy will benefit from a strength training exercise program aimed at reducing her risk of falls and through activities that improve balance and mobility.
- Mrs. Levy may be distracted by a table game at the nurses' station that she can work on until she is ready to go back to her room. A favorite videotape or music on a headset may help her go back to sleep. She also may be comforted and distracted by an offer to polish her fingernails or brush her hair.

- Mrs. Levy is unlikely to be able to identify her recently created art projects as hers. If she insists that you take her name off her artwork, simply do it and say that you like the particular piece and that you are sorry to have upset her.
- Mrs. Levy might respond well to time spent with a dog or other pet.
- Provide her with a repetitive work task. Sorting a silverware drawer, tearing newspaper for the craft room, shining silver, winding yarn, rolling pennies for the bank, or cutting coupons are several jobs that can be done regularly.

Environmental Strategies

- Take any items from her room that increase her risk of falls or threaten her security.
- Set the dining room table with placecards to reassure her that she is expected and a legitimate diner.
- Find a room or area close to her room that feels "safe" to her and take her there to rest after the frustration caused by the little people in her room. Tell her this is a room for peace and quiet.
- Make sure the little people are not the result of glare from a street lamp and the bugs are not a pattern in the floor design.

Tip Checklist

1. Reassure Mrs. Levy with understanding and concern in response to her hallucinations or delusions. Make sure they are not a result of something in the environment.
2. Do not remind residents that a beloved family member is dead.
3. Some residents will need to stay up at night and sleep later in the morning.

INAPPROPRIATE SOCIAL BEHAVIOR

"Does she have no shame?"

Mrs. Paisley, a 65-year-old resident with a diagnosis of Pick's Disease, had run a fancy hotel restaurant with her husband. Now she undresses without closing the door to her room, dresses sloppily, eats food off other people's plates, and chases her devoted husband from the facility with shouts of "Go to hell!" Mrs. Paisley calls a dignified older resident "the rich bitch" and regularly refers to nurse assistants as "poor white trash," regardless of their race. But the next minute, she will be seen following her favorite assistant, Patience, through the facility and even into the staff bathroom. She begs Patience to "Let me go home with you. I promise to be good." She becomes furious when Patience attends to other residents, insisting that they are old and crippled and not as cute as she is. Mrs. Paisley also flirts with other women's husbands and once asked a male visitor, who had just greeted her pleasantly, if he wanted to see "her boobies." Today, Mrs. Paisley was found in bed with an older married male resident who has AD. They were both naked.

What's Going On?

Pick's Disease is a frontotemporal dementia. Residents with this illness are often younger than residents with other dementias, and their changes in behavior and ability to control impulses are more noticeable than their memory problems. Extremes are common with Pick's Disease, and residents are described as being really sweet one minute and outrageous the next. Sometimes, they act uncharacteristically silly. Their behavior may look and even sound childish, but treating them like children only makes it worse. Mrs. Paisley cannot resist saying and doing whatever comes into her head. It has nothing to do with any delayed secret or long-standing wish to rebel or "cut loose." This is not necessarily her true self coming out.

Her behavior changes make it hard for her husband to know which Mrs. Paisley he will meet each day. Her cursing and tactless behavior obviously embarrass him. Her immodest behavior and poor table manners are a result of her lost awareness of where she is and what is public and private. Mrs. Paisley's affection for Patience is an attempt to find comfort and reassurance. She feels safe with Patience, perhaps like she felt as a little girl. Mrs. Paisley believes that Patience will protect her. But needing Patience also makes Mrs. Paisley mad about not being able to control her.

Mrs. Paisley has the same needs for sexual intimacy and comfort as she probably had before. But like most nursing facility residents, she has fewer acceptable ways to meet those needs. Residents with dementia may display affection by holding hands, kissing, or hugging other residents or visitors and this may meet mutual needs for companionship. Mrs. Paisley may also feel a need for sexual stimulation and may masturbate in public, often because there is so little opportunity for privacy. It is not unusual for residents with memory disorders to make unwanted verbal or physical advances, grabbing or touching staff or other residents, and even disrobing or showing off their genitals in public.

Strategies That Work

Prevention Tips

Spouses should receive information at admission about what to expect from people with this condition. A matter-of-fact information session lets families know that loss of inhibition and misidentification of other residents as spouses causes a variety of uncomfortable and unusual behaviors, some of which are sexual. When educated about possible inappropriate comments or behaviors in advance, spouses may be more comfortable during visits. Families should be told that the need for sexual expression is normal for adults her age, regardless of medical conditions, but that the facility will do its best to protect residents and visitors from injury or embarrassment. Let Mr. Paisley know that if his wife's inappropriate behavior becomes a problem for other residents or visitors, a meeting with his wife's doctor, nursing staff, and other involved parties, including an ombudsman or ethics committee, will be held to develop a plan that meets Mrs. Paisley's and the staff's needs, preferences, and capacities. Ideally, an admission assessment has identified general information about her relationship history and intimacy styles and any behavioral excesses of a sexual nature that occurred before admission.

Mrs. Paisley's inappropriate behaviors should be documented in the chart. It may not be necessary to inform her husband about her showing "her boobies" because it was stopped and redirected successfully by staff. No one was hurt or especially distressed. All that is needed is to reassure the visitor that some behavior is unpredictable, but that the staff understands his discomfort and will try to help Mrs. Paisley avoid causing further discomfort to others. When Mrs. Paisley is found naked in bed with another resident, this behavior must be documented in both residents' charts, families and physicians must be notified, and a meeting should be held to determine how to handle the behavior.

Communicating With Mrs. Paisley

Patience needs to maintain a friendly but firm response to Mrs. Paisley. When Mrs. Paisley becomes demanding, Patience can just remark, "No rest for the weary, I guess." She should not blame, reason, or confront Mrs. Paisley about her outrageous behavior. She should acknowledge her and help her feel like they understand each other. When Patience needs a break from Mrs. Paisley, she might say, "I know where to find you. I'll come when you need me. I bet you'll enjoy sitting with Mrs. Thomas for a minute until I'm ready for you." When Patience returns, she is likely to hear Mrs. Paisley telling Mrs. Thomas that Patience walked off on her just like all the unreliable people around here. That's when staff's sense of humor and tolerance for bizarre confusion will be essential.

Also, staff need to understand that Mrs. Paisley's tactless insults do not indicate real prejudice or displeasure with any one person. She is upset with her situation and cannot control her response to it. Try not to respond to insults. She may stop if her words do not arouse attention. On the other hand, excessively polite responses, such as "please" or "yes, ma'am," may trigger Mrs. Paisley's automatic hostess behavior.

When Mrs. Paisley tries to flash male visitors, calmly tell Mrs. Paisley that you see that she wants your help with her shirt, and rebutton it for her. She really is seeking attention, and by helping her with her shirt, you are offering her that attention. Give her a hug, covering her exposed front from view, and compliment her on her "great hugs." Diversion or distraction in a calm, reassuring, and normal sounding voice works best. Perhaps a medication is making her sexual feelings more difficult to control.

It is important to find stimulating sensory approaches to meet Mrs. Paisley's needs for intimacy and touch in more acceptable ways, such as massaging her hand, giving her a back rub, or having her use the whirlpool. Aromatherapy or a stuffed animal are other ways to meet her sensory needs. Reassure Mr. Paisley that you will try to keep his wife from being embarrassed. Suggest that he must miss her attention now that she is so focused on herself. Let him know you will not judge him or their relationship on the basis of her present behavior.

When she takes others' food, do not punish or scold Mrs. Paisley. Just say she must be hungry today, and give the other resident a fresh plate of food. To help her recognize her own meal, provide Mrs. Paisley with a unique-looking plate, such as one with a floral design or unbreakable china.

Activities Of Daily Living

1. Mrs. Paisley may behave more acceptably if she is dressed in clothing that fastens in the back, making it more difficult for her to disrobe in public.
2. Consider giving Mrs. Paisley a "fanny pack" with favorite snacks or items she can fondle or hold. Unzipping and rezipping the bag may be a good substitute for disrobing.
3. Bathing should provide an opportunity for pampering. Talk about the pleasurable aspects of bathing and use feminine luxury items to enhance her sensory experience.
4. Eating and mealtime activities should be highlighted to remind Mrs. Paisley of her former career and the niceties that go along with fine dining.
5. Attention to privacy should be accentuated in providing personal care. If she grabs at staff in a sexual way, she should be given something for the grabbing hand to hold and told, "This is for your hand. Please stop grabbing."
6. Mrs. Paisley should be given plenty of time and opportunity to apply makeup and skin care lotions, put on jewelry, and fix her hair—all day if necessary. Appointments with a hairdresser would be a nice treat.

Activities

- Patience will need to accompany Mrs. Paisley to activities at first. She can introduce her to activities with comments like, "Let's see what's going on. I smell cookies baking." If Mrs. Paisley is insulting, tactless, or inappropriate in small group activities, she will need guidance and supervision for structured individual activities that she can work on in her room.
- Mrs. Paisley might benefit from a behavior box approach. This is a box of items that remind her of familiar activities. Her box

might contain a restaurant ledger or receipt book, grocery lists, or a wipe-off board with tables outlined for waiter assignments.

• A special collection of videotapes and a bedroom videocassette recorder (VCR) could keep her occupied sometimes. Her husband can tape favorite old television shows, movies, or cooking shows that can be replayed when she needs private time.

• Speakers and guest performers should be warned that it is nothing personal if Mrs. Paisley puts down their efforts. Tell the visitor, "She's not very happy with herself right now, but I think she enjoys your program. Please do not take it personally."

• Mrs. Paisley would benefit from activities that focus on her appearance—spending extra time on facials or selecting perfume.

• Mrs. Paisley is young and vigorous and needs appropriate exercise programs and activities. Her sexual energy can be redirected to vigorous appropriate exercise.

• Mrs. Paisley may enjoy dressing and undressing a doll in multiple layers of clothing.

• Mrs. Paisley may enjoy fashion magazines or old romance movies on video.

Environmental Strategies

Mrs. Paisley may find a body pillow comforting in bed. Often, hypersexual female residents will use potentially injurious objects to stimulate themselves, and a soft large object is much safer. She also may find mirrors reassuring. Her room should offer reminders of her successful career and opportunities to rearrange things.

Tip Checklist

1. Calmly cover up a resident who is disrobing.
2. Try massage, body pillows, or facials for residents who exhibit inappropriate sexual behavior.
3. Remember that the disease—not the resident—is responsible for the behavior. Continue to treat the resident with kindness and respect.

THE SUNDOWNING EFFECT

"Packin' it up for tonight's gig"

Mr. James, a 70-year-old newly admitted resident with AD and vascular dementia, is social most of the time, but he becomes very irritable during afternoon shift change. He paces, pulls at his clothes, and even becomes verbally abusive with his new friend, whom he calls his "buddy from the club." He enjoys the sunroom for most of the day, but resists going with a staff member and group to the outdoor area in the late afternoon. Instead, he complains that he is already late and "the club patrons won't wait for nobody." Mr. James, a former jazz pianist, has been divorced several times, and has a daughter, Hope, who visits regularly, often with her dog, Cajun.

His agitation grows after dark. He packs and unpacks his clothes in plastic bags for his next road trip. He calls his daughter for a ride to the club, and when he starts crying about never missing a gig, she begs the staff to offer him a sedative. She says she cannot stand to see her formerly confident, celebrity dad reduced to this. He is disrupting the staff and upsetting the other residents, particularly his passive friend, whose friendship has been the key to his adjustment at the facility.

What's Going On?

People with brain disorders become more confused, restless, and insecure late in the day, and especially after dark. This happens whether they are living at home or in a facility, but often it is worse after a move or change in routines. They feel threatened and may try to return to a more familiar and reassuring place, whether it is "Mama's" or a job. Repetitive, anxious packing behaviors are quite common, even at home. When residents become agitated late in the day, their sleep/wake cycles are disrupted and they may be more demanding, restless, confused, impulsive, suspicious, or disoriented and may even see, hear, or believe things that are not real. Attention span and concentration become even more limited. This late-afternoon distress is called sundowning.

Although there are many possible explanations for sundowning, a likely suspect is fatigue. Late in the day, many residents become exhausted from trying to keep up with a strange environment. In addition, the increased activity of shift change or decreased light in the late afternoon may frighten residents and increase their agitation and frustration. Sometimes, other residents and staff are running out of steam, and the resident may be responding to the nonverbal cues in the environment. The sundowning behavior may be a response to one particular person in the environment or being asked to do something that is too complex.

Can Sundowning Be Prevented?

Identifying triggers to sundowning behaviors requires real detective work. Some residents may be upset by late afternoon programming on television. They may feel crowded or closed in by the shorter days and longer periods of dark in the winter. Afternoon agitation also may be a response to caffeine, hunger, uncomfortable clothing, or a fruitless search for the bathroom. Some strategies to try to avoid the sundowning effect can include:

- Making sure the resident has frequent brief rests in his room to restore his composure.
- Turning off loud or upsetting television shows in the late afternoon.
- Observing what happens just before the resident starts to become upset.
- Reducing expectations late in the day.
- Increasing lighting or closing draperies if late afternoon light

creates confusing shadows.
- Increasing fluid intake throughout the day.
- Checking medications for dosing, timing, interactions, or side effects.
- Removing reminders of travel, such as suitcases and plastic bags.
- Implementing a cocktail hour at the facility with nonalcoholic sparkling drinks and appropriate snacks.

Strategies That Work

Communicating With Mr. James

Helping Mr. James stay calm in the late afternoon is staff's greatest challenge. Distractions may help. Possible distractions for Mr. James might include reminding him that he has time to relax before the next gig; getting him to tell you about his last gig; or offering reassurance, such as, "You can relax tonight—it's Sunday and the club is closed. The club knows you would never let them down." These distraction techniques may help Mr. James settle down. Do not blatantly lie when using distractions, such as telling an agitated resident that her mother—who died decades ago—will be here shortly. It is better to encourage the resident to reminisce about her mother instead.

Other tips include walking with Mr. James and listening for clues—such as when he has a visible angry response when he passes one particular female resident in the hall. The woman keeps saying, "Get outta here," and Mr. James mumbles, "There she is again. She never lets up." Perhaps encounters with this resident set him off. Later you may learn from Hope that her father said the same thing about one of his ex-wives who complained that he didn't earn enough money. He may think she is the ex-wife or her comments may just remind him of not living up to expectations. In addition, tell him that you understand he is a night owl and respect his preferences.

Activities Of Daily Living

1. Try adjusting Mr. James's routine so he can get up later in the morning, and offer him a late supper before he goes to sleep at a later hour at night.
2. Maybe listening to music or having a nonalcoholic beer before dinner would stimulate his appetite. Try suggesting that all meals and drinks are covered in his "club membership."
3. Make sure Mr. James is kept away from the resident who upsets him. She may be setting the stage for his increased agitation if he thinks she is critical of him.
4. Mr. James needs reminders and help using the toilet. Once positioned, give him as much privacy as possible by moving out of his line of vision.
5. If Mr. James was used to bathing late in the afternoon before work, that routine might divert him from his rush to pack and get on the road. Tell him what you are doing and what he needs to do one step at a time. Singing or listening to music during bathing may help him relax.

Activities

• Make sure Mr. James is well supplied with his favorite jazz tapes. Just before the usual time his agitation escalates in the late afternoon, take him to his room, put on a tape, and ask if he could listen to it and make suggestions for the dinner music for the evening.
• Mr. James enjoys his visits with Cajun. If Hope cannot bring her dog each afternoon, perhaps a pet therapy dog could be brought to the facility in the late afternoon to visit with the residents. Another dog would provide a comparison and an outlet for touching and affection as well as something to talk about and take care of.
• Mr. James needs things to pack. Tell him you need his help or ask him to show you how to pack, sort, or carry out the recycling.

He can be asked to pack or sort donated records or jazz tapes for the facility music room.

- Mr. James needs time apart from his buddy until he is ready to greet him again as a long-lost friend. Try to arrange separate activities for them in the late afternoon.
- Mr. James should be encouraged to play a piano or keyboard if that still pleases him. Some accomplished musicians become frustrated when they realize they are no longer able to play like they used to. An alternative would be to have someone else play and ask him to help determine if the piano needs tuning or which keys are out of tune.
- Try to arrange brief outings to jazz concerts with his daughter or ask his daughter to encourage his club friends to visit and reminisce with him. Let them know that "talking shop" about the old days on the road might bring moments of pleasure even if it does not reduce his agitation completely. Try to bring "club music" entertainment to the facility and have Mr. James's career acknowledged at the performance.
- Mr. James spent much of his career composing music. Giving him music composition sheets may prompt his memory and provide an adult activity to work on.
- Mr. James could be asked to join a bell ringers, percussion, or drummers group—sometimes it is more fun and less threatening to try a new instrument like a tambourine or cymbal.
- Mr. James may need more structured evening activities like dances or parties after supper. If no planned activities are possible, he could be asked to help deliver items to rooms or check that lights are on and working throughout the unit.
- If Mr. James is really agitated, he needs a physical activity that releases some of that energy. Consider kicking a beach ball, batting a balloon back and forth, bean bag toss, or tearing newspaper into sheets to use for Cajun's longer visits to the facility. Doing these things with his buddy might make them more fun.

Environmental Strategies

- Mr. James's room should reflect his career success and recognition, unless those memories are contributing to his agitation about leaving for the club. Having a room decorated like a jazz club may not be conducive to sleep or personal care or may even stimulate his desire for a cigarette. If so, perhaps a corner of a sitting room could be decorated to look like a nightclub, with round tables and a piano.
- Mr. James has a favorite collection of old sheet music that could be displayed prominently in his room. If a small space is available in a common area, convert it to a music room. Old music boxes and instruments can be stored there as well as old wind-up radios and victrolas.
- Mr. James needs to be separated from people who trigger his agitation or threats at times during the day when he is more likely to become agitated. You may learn that his agitation in the late afternoon is not triggered by the woman who looks like his ex-wife, but by his late afternoon trips down the elevator. Perhaps he can be escorted down a stairwell instead.

Tip Checklist

1. Offer frequent breaks during the day to reduce fatigue.
2. Separate residents who seem to upset each other, especially during the late afternoon.
3. Offer quiet time in his room in the late afternoon to limit his agitation.

CATASTROPHIC REACTIONS

"It's all your fault!"

Mrs. Robins is a tiny, 82-year-old widow with a recent diagnosis of AD. She had been the model minister's wife and is now living in a church-run assisted living facility. She keeps to herself and never asks for help. She has no visitors. The church facility is far from her home church, and her only son is a missionary in Africa. Mrs. Robins refuses to participate in activities, insisting that her church duties keep her busy enough. After months of coaxing, she has agreed to help "bake" cookies to give to children coming to sing Christmas carols. A program staff person stops by to tell her they are ready to bake. Mrs. Robins has been "getting ready" to leave her room all morning, but has not made much progress. When the staff person offers to help her dress, Mrs. Robins yells, "No! Get away from me! I've been saved and I don't need help from sinners." But Mrs. Robins shows up in the baking room moments later and sweetly takes an offered apron. She is chatting with another resident, stirring her bowl, when she sees that flour has been spilled on the counter. Suddenly, she screams at the resident next to her, "Now look what you've done. I try to do my Christian duty and you ruin everything. Lord save me." She stomps out of the room.

What's Going On?

Catastrophic reaction is a term used to describe the behavior of people with brain disorders when a situation overwhelms their ability to think and react appropriately. Mrs. Robins is overwhelmed and defensive and becomes stubborn, critical, or overly emotional—all out of proportion to the incident. Catastrophic reactions can be set off by any number of things, including:

• Being asked several questions at once, especially "why" questions.

- Feelings of insecurity, perhaps from feeling lost or left alone.
- Small mishaps like spilled milk or missed ingredients.
- Too many strange people in a new place with new sights and sounds.
- Television or radio shows that she has trouble separating from reality. She may think she is the character who is attacked by sinners after watching religious programming.
- Feeling criticized or contradicted; having an argument.
- An overstimulating, noisy, crowded, or unpredictable environment that is misjudged or misinterpreted.
- Tense, irritated, rushed, or impatient staff members.
- A sense of failure in completing a task she once regarded as simple, such as baking. Because Mrs. Robins' judgment is impaired, she cannot evaluate the seriousness of any minor mistake in baking.

Preventing Outbursts

- Change or reduce expectations and limit activities to those that guarantee success, such as being a baking taster.
- Limit decision making. Rather than ask if she wants to bake, ask her if she wants to do the mixing or help with decorating the cookies.
- Do not ask questions about why she is upset. Stay calm and help her leave a group activity until she is more composed. Reassure or support her until she feels better. She's probably too upset to know or say what's wrong.
- Offer guidance one step at a time. Repeat suggestions word-for-word if she does not follow through.
- Distract her gradually with something new. Do not remind her that she lost control and did something embarrassing. Let forgetting work for her self-esteem.
- Suggest to visitors that they keep visits calm and simple.
- Try to identify what might be triggering Mrs. Robins' fear of sinners. The chaplain learned that Mrs. Robins' husband had

been a missionary and that African villagers had threatened the family. Mrs. Robins may be frightened of staff or residents who are African American.

Strategies That Work

Communicating With Mrs. Robins

Mrs. Robins may need to determine if you are "like her." She may repetitively ask, "Are you saved?" You can say, "Yes, ma'am," or "I know you are saved by the grace of your presence." Either one would reassure Mrs. Robins that you are a "safe" person. Seek Mrs. Robins' counsel in questions of faith. There are no right answers but she will be reassured by your interest in her all-consuming thoughts. Start every conversation with, "I'm sorry to bother you when you are busy with your church work, but I could use your help with..." Let her know that you think she is a good woman who has done her Christian duty.

After an outburst, give her time alone to compose herself by suggesting that you will check back with her later. Apologize for upsetting her. Just say, "I'm terribly sorry, Mrs. Robins. I shouldn't have interrupted you." She must believe that she has the right to say "no" and to determine her best time to participate in group or social activities. In group activities, always ask if she has time to help with one of two acceptable choices. Perhaps the first time she participates in baking, she could be the critic who offers suggestions about which ingredients might be added next time.

African American staff must be told about her traumatic past experience and reminded that they should not take her verbal abuse personally. Mrs. Robins feels alone among "foreigners in a foreign land." Find ways to help her feel connected to someone—a staff person from the same denomination, a chaplain with a similar history, or a local children's Sunday School class that can "adopt" her for visits or special attention at holidays.

Activities Of Daily Living

1. Tell Mrs. Robins what you are doing and why, and offer one-step guidance with dressing. For instance, tell her, "I am helping with the buttons on the back of your blouse. Would you like me to leave the top button open?"
2. Adapt her clothing so she can do more for herself. Lay clothing out in the order it will be put on. Limit choices in her closet or drawers.
3. Keep her routines as structured, orderly, and predictable as possible. If she seems to be most cooperative with one staff member, try consistent assignment.
4. Get her to bathe by telling her that tomorrow is Sunday and she will want to be fresh for church.
5. Sing her favorite hymns or ask her to recite her favorite psalms as you help her with dressing or bathing.
6. Offer her an opportunity to ask the blessing at her table or to host her table. Always remind her that the church family takes care of dedicated members like her.
7. Play peaceful or joyful church music during personal care.

Activities

Avoid messy activities that might upset Mrs. Robins. Some residents become upset during baking if they believe it is too unpredictable or out of control. In addition, previous hobbies and interests may not be pleasant now.

Observe what she does with her time alone and try to incorporate activities that build on that. Find a way to include sweets, snacks, or treats at the end of any activity. It will leave a pleasant memory if only for a brief time. Mrs. Robins may retain better control with small group activities. Or, leave cross-stitch magazines in her room and ask her to pick out her favorites.

To capitalize on her spiritual needs, give her a book of psalms to carry with her as a security object. Ask the chaplain to prepare a visiting kit for her of familiar and comforting religious items and reminders, or form a Bible study or small prayer group and let her select the content. In addition, be sure that she is taken to church, chapel services, choir sings, and a variety of activities that will not require her active leadership. The familiarity may be comforting. Never ask her to do leisure or playful activities on Sundays. In addition, supervise her access to religious programming—some preaching on the "wages of sin" may be upsetting her.

Environmental Strategies

- Personalize Mrs. Robins' room with mementos of her success, such as pictures of her with her Sunday school classes.
- A guardian angel statue or painting may be more reassuring than a crucifix.
- If she likes to keep things neat and orderly, help her put her things away or give her containers to keep her things in.

Tip Checklist

1. Give residents a graceful way to decline participation in activities that frustrate them.
2. Build on activities that a resident does on her own, or does well.
3. Offer opportunities for residents to recite remembered blessings or poems from childhood.

EARLY ONSET ALZHEIMER'S

"Thank you, but I won't be staying"

Mrs. Barton, a 52-year-old wife and mother, has just been admitted to an Alzheimer's unit. Her visibly shaken family dropped her off and left. She is attractive but looks intense and on guard. Staff have been unable to draw her out of her private room, and she missed lunch. She keeps telling staff, "Thank you, but I won't be staying." She has refused to change clothes and insists, "There has been a terrible mistake." She has asked to call the police.

What's Going On?

Mr. Barton knew that his wife would have a difficult adjustment to a facility caring primarily for older people, but he believed his daughters deserved relief from the chaos of the last two years at home. Even so, he and his daughters were too overwhelmed to offer any information about Mrs. Barton at admission, such as her interests or abilities. In addition, Mr. Barton believed he should minimize his wife's difficulties with personal care and her behavioral outbursts to "protect" her and their family from further embarrassment. Mrs. Barton was admitted just before her husband left town on business and her daughters were reluctant to visit without him. Staff were not sure how to respond to this woman who looked so young and seemed so in control.

Mrs. Barton still has a good vocabulary, although she repeats the same words often. She sounds much better than she actually functions because she fills in the blanks in her memory with repetitive but incorrect information that seems to make sense. It is likely that Mrs. Barton is resistive because she is not sure what is expected of her and she does not want to make a mistake.

While the characteristics of Mrs. Barton's AD are similar to those of older residents with the disease, her family was completely unprepared to deal with her diagnosis and behavior changes. As a result, they were reluctant to share stories about her or provide a list of her interests and abilities. Staff only know she was diagnosed with AD three years ago. Her admission forms indicate that she is independent in ADLs, but it is possible that her husband simply denied her disability. Maybe she is resistive because she does not know what is expected of her or she is afraid of making a mistake. Without initial family support and information, staff will need to get to know Mrs. Barton on their own to learn how to work with her.

If possible, it will be helpful if a staff member can convince Mr. Barton that his knowledge of his wife's abilities and disabilities are invaluable in helping staff adapt to her needs and preferences. Perhaps someone else who knows her well could help the staff understand and respond to her in ways that she finds reassuring (*see Chapter Four for helping families adjust*).

Soon after admission, Mrs. Barton's cousin comes to visit and privately fills in the staff on the blanks in Mrs. Barton's history. Her parents ran a jewelry store, and Mrs. Barton joined their business as a designer until the neighborhood changed and there were frequent robberies. Her father was shot and killed during a robbery. The cousin thinks that Mrs. Barton has never felt safe since the store robberies, and her last vivid memory is that you call police when you are in trouble. The cousin thinks Mrs. Barton is more impaired in ADLs than her husband is willing to admit. She had stopped changing clothes prior to her admission and had difficulty fixing her hair.

Strategies That Work

Communicating With Mrs. Barton

To try to gain Mrs. Barton's trust, a staff member should knock on her door and ask permission to visit. When she says, "Thank you, but I won't be staying," the staff member can say, "I understand that. I just want to get to know you while I can. May I sit over here next to your picture?" Ask about the picture of her with her parents. What were they doing? What did her parents call her? At that, she brightens up and says without hesitation, "Rosie." Talk about how she got that nickname. You share a laugh and tell her that you, too, had a childhood name. Now you have something in common. Do not ask her to do anything on this first visit. Make it a friendly visit.

When she starts to talk about the police again, say, "I'm thirsty—please join me for a cup of tea. There's another Rosie down the hall that I would love for you to meet." If she protests that she has to wait for the police, tell her that other people in the building will know where she is if anyone is looking for her. This is your chance to introduce her to at least one other resident, observe her eating skills, and begin to build trust.

Be honest with her about how hard it is to face so many changes. Encourage her that with time, you will learn each other's ways and she will relax and feel safer. As the staff becomes familiar with her retained skills and interests, they can create an abilities-focused plan that will not just keep her busy, but will encourage her to be a part of a community where people have fun and help each other.

Communicating With Mrs. Barton's Family

Mr. Barton may be overwhelmed with his new responsibilities of raising his daughters alone and dealing with the family's grief. He may feel like he is failing everyone and everything at once while everyone is depending on him. It is difficult for him to see his wife so changed and so unconcerned about him. He tells the staff that his wife managed her business, the house, and the family, and he never noticed what she did until she could no longer explain it to him. He wants to hide from the accusing or sad looks of his family.

Mr. Barton needs staff to demonstrate interest and concern for him before he will be able to help staff with his wife. Staff can ask him how he met his wife or how they started working together. He may relax if he is asked "normal" questions before being asked about her current functioning and behavior. Remind him that the easiest way for staff to help her is for staff to learn about her through him.

Suggest a good time for him to visit when key staff are available to speak with him. Help him find ways to involve his daughters with their mother without requiring them to visit. Teens often are more relaxed when accompanying a resident on outings rather than visiting within the facility.

Activities Of Daily Living

Upon returning to her room, staff can remark to Mrs. Barton that she must be tired from today's travel. Suggest that she may want to change into something more comfortable. Perhaps she would like to use the bathroom first. While she is in the bathroom, pull two nightgowns from her suitcases and when she comes out, ask which she prefers. If she looks startled or resistant, you may suggest that she wants to take her jewelry off first and you can help with that. Calmly and slowly assist her out of her clothes, and ask if you may hang them up "just for now." Observe how she manages her clothing and offer only one-step cues as needed. Take it slow. Once in her nightclothes, she may be more comfortable sitting in a chair before getting into bed. Tell her there's no harm in dozing off in front of the television. Offer her some privacy and one of her magazines from home, but reassure her that you will check in to see if she needs anything later.

Mrs. Barton needs to establish a predictable routine. Everyone who assists her should help her in the same way. Always ask her to help you and make sure she does as much as she can for herself. Later on, her family may want to bring clothing that is easier to get on and off.

Mrs. Barton's jewelry is an important connection to her past. Find ways to talk about jewelry while assisting her. Perhaps you can help her put away her jewelry first and gradually organize the rest of her clothing. Present guided choices between two acceptable storage places and always ask her preferences—is this how you like your closet?

Mrs. Barton should be "invited" to meals with another resident, pointing out things they have in common. She should be routinely escorted to meals until she learns her way.

Assume bathing will be a struggle at first. Ask her if she prefers baths or showers. If she resists, just calmly tell her it is part of the "service" that her family requested. Offer her as much privacy as she can handle and let her relax in the bathtub before washing up. If she brought shampoo from home, comment on what good taste she has. Talk about hairstyles and how many she has tried. Compliment her at every opportunity and suggest that the other residents might like to see how nice she looks when she is done.

Mrs. Barton has had many recent changes. Once she can depend on a routine and develop a sense of place, she will relax and feel safer. As the staff get to know her retained skills and interests, they can create an abilities-focused plan for her and help her become part of the facility community.

Activities

Mrs. Barton will not join any activity on her own and probably will refuse all invitations. Let her say "no" a few times. Then invite her to a small women's coffee group. Mrs. Barton can be asked to go through a box of costume jewelry and help decide what to keep and how to decide which jewelry goes together.

She may need more one-on-one time with another resident, volunteer, or staff member who can accompany her to activities where she will meet other residents. Mrs. Barton needs a special identity within the facility, whether it is as "Rosie," the jewelry lady, or as a fashion consultant. She also needs a way to connect with other residents or staff to feel like she belongs.

Her cousin has agreed to take Mrs. Barton to her regular hairdresser weekly as a special outing with lunch. Mrs. Barton needs time with someone who knew her childhood and parents and remembers the stories of their mutual past. Mrs. Barton does not remember her cousin's name but knows she is family and always returns from these outings more relaxed and happy.

Staff learn that Mrs. Barton has won golf trophies. She loves wearing her golf clothes to exercise programs in the facility. She is asked to demonstrate "her swing" for the other residents and golf becomes another way to engage Mrs. Barton in conversations with staff, residents, and visitors.

In addition, Mrs. Barton is encouraged to help water plants and clip herbs for supper. When she appears in the dining room looking for a cup of tea, she is often given some napkins to fold for supper, a task she seems to enjoy. Repetitive tasks seem to comfort her when she is upset and staff encourage her to sit in the dining room or the sunroom when she is having a rough day or time. Because she enjoys brief outings, she is included in occasional small group outings with staff to a botanical garden and a putting green.

Environmental Strategies

Mrs. Barton's room should be personalized to reflect her interests and to show off her trophies. Pictures from her childhood and golfing should be brought in. To keep track of important events, Mrs. Barton should be given her own calendar with the weekly outing prominently displayed along with other events. She may enjoy crossing off each day during morning care and discussing the number of days until her next outing. She may also like to work on items from a box of costume jewelry in her room.

You can tell when residents with Alzheimer's are doing better. Mrs. Barton will relax and you will see more of her sense of humor. She will talk less about her need for the police and more about herself. She will start asking for what she wants rather than just refusing to participate. She will talk more openly and will find new friends on her own. She will show more pride in herself, more warmth, and maybe even affection with people she likes, whether they look "old" to her or not. Her creativity and pleasure with what she does in any activity (whether dressing or an arts program) will let you know that she feels at home and among friends.

Tip Checklist

1. Younger residents with AD exhibit the same behavioral characteristics as older people with AD. However, their families may have a more difficult time coming to terms with the diagnosis and may not offer a lot of support.
2. Younger residents should be acknowledged as younger—and treated by staff as such.
3. Use "just for now" approaches with residents who insist they are leaving soon.

END-OF-LIFE CARE

"Help me, help me"

Mrs. Reston is a 93-year-old widow who has lived in a skilled nursing facility for the last 10 years with a diagnosis of AD. She has outlived most of her family, but her 70-year-old daughter, Frances, visits regularly. Frances has health care power of attorney. Mrs. Reston had a living will and a "do not resuscitate" order (now called "allow natural death") when she entered the facility, and Mrs. Reston had expressed strong negative feelings about feeding tubes in her living will and to her daughter after watching her husband die with a feeding tube. Mrs. Reston weighs 87 pounds; she has not walked since a fall months ago, has occasional seizures, and sleeps much of the time. When she is awake, she pulls at her blankets, cries, moans, grunts, and calls out incessantly, "Help me, help me."

Mrs. Reston has frequent infections and fevers and with each medical event, Frances rushes over and asks why the staff is not helping her mother. Frances thinks staff are neglecting her mother because she has run out of money. Frances also gathers her church prayer group around her mother's bed regularly, which seems to upset Mrs. Reston even more. Mrs. Reston is difficult to feed, often clamping her jaws shut around the spoon or knocking the food off the spoon with her good arm. She screams even louder when she is repositioned. She calls out whenever staff leave the room.

What's Going On?

Families want to know what to expect and how to respond to the unique needs of people with AD nearing death. At the end of life, some events are fairly consistent. Most people with Alzheimer's forget how to walk at some point or may just fall when walking. It is hard for them to relearn to walk after a fall or to cooperate with rehabilitation efforts. Everyone with end-stage Alzheimer's becomes incontinent of bladder and bowel. Immobility and incontinence make people vulnerable to frequent infections. At the end of life, residents with Alzheimer's eat and drink less. Swallowing problems and choking are common. With inadequate nutrition and hydration, the skin becomes thin and breaks down easily.

Most people with Alzheimer's sleep more at the end of life or withdraw by closing their eyes. Never assume that people like this are sleeping or cannot hear. Restless repetitive movements like pulling at a sheet and repetitive calling out, sometimes called disruptive vocalizations, are also common. Dying people, regardless of their diagnosis, frequently have visions and talk or call out to people long dead. As dying Alzheimer's residents go back in time, they commonly summon up the earliest memories of security—their mother.

Changes in breathing patterns or irregular shallow breathing patterns may cause a moaning-like sound when these residents exhale. Congestion is common when weakness makes it impossible to cough up secretions. There are frequent changes in temperature and skin color, especially around the hands and feet. Some people with Alzheimer's develop seizures at the end, and they may become completely unresponsive in the last few days.

Strategies That Work

Minimizing Distress And Discomfort

- Progression of the disease is inevitable, but good comfort care, or palliative care, can improve the quality of living and dying. A resident dying with Alzheimer's presents an opportunity to do something. It is not the time to withdraw, abandon, or "let nature take its course." Offer hope and extra one-on-one time. Reminders of your affection, without being unrealistically optimistic about Mrs. Reston's recovery, can help to soothe and calm her. Hope is based on confidence in your ability to care for and about her, not cure her.

- Focus on meeting Frances's needs for reassurance. Teach her how to soothe and comfort her mother, talking softly, reassuring her, stroking her hand, and praying. Remind Frances that her presence is what is really important now.
- Offer frequent, small amounts of thickened liquids, pureed items, or protein and calorie-enhanced foods, and limit these to foods that Mrs. Reston likes. Some residents smack their lips or otherwise let you know that one food or drink is particularly appealing. Some residents develop strong sucking needs and do better with flexible straws or frozen treats.
- Proper positioning can reduce choking. Never force feed or pry open a resident's mouth when it is clamped shut. However, if the resident has something in her mouth and has not swallowed, try gently stroking the side of her cheek. If the resident cannot swallow, remove the food from her mouth and prop up her head for a short time.
- If she refuses all fluids, use glycerin swabs on her mouth to keep her lips moist.
- Encourage Frances to ask prayer group members to come individually to provide one-to-one attention and a "healing presence."
- Reposition and change pads frequently to avoid use of disposable adult undergarments.
- Treat constipation or diarrhea with diet changes as needed. Suggest evaluation for pain if she screams, squirms, or frowns when repositioned.
- When she is having breathing problems, try elevating her head or turning her face to the side. Added oxygen may make her more comfortable if she can tolerate it.
- Ask for a consultation from or referral to hospice. Frances may need reassurance of their expertise and availability. Hospice adds the value of knowledgeable staff experienced in pain management and end-of-life care. Frances also may need permission to let go and not rush to the bedside with each change in condition. A

trained counselor can help her decide if visiting is helping or making things harder for her. The hospice chaplain could help Frances and provide another healing presence for Mrs. Reston.

Communicating With Mrs. Reston And Frances

To help Mrs. Reston, staff and visitors should be encouraged to hold her hand gently, talk reassuringly, repeat her favorite prayers, talk about her "mama," and let her know that people are there for her. Tell her what you are doing before you do it. Give her time to respond. Ask her what hurts or touch where you think it hurts and ask her if that is the place. Then ask her if what you are doing is making her feel better.

Suggest that Frances talk to her mother about how much she is loved and how she made a difference in her life. Suggest that Frances recite favorite poems, stories, prayers, or hymns with her mother. Remind Frances of her important role as Mrs. Reston's memory. In addition, encourage Frances to ask the doctor about options for treatment of infections, feeding, hydration, and the benefits and risks of aggressive diagnosis and treatment in a hospital. Assure Frances that staff will provide dignified personal care and comfort regardless of treatment decisions.

Finally, after she dies, allow Frances to have time with Mrs. Reston's body, if she desires, before it is moved. Ask her if she would like staff to call someone to be with her. Staff may unknowingly offer too much privacy to family members who need a comforting staff presence when they feel sad or helpless. Offer a memorial service at the facility for staff, families, residents, and Frances's prayer group. Be sure everyone has the opportunity to tell Frances what her mother meant to them on a personal level. Call Frances within a month after the death to let her know that you are thinking of her and you know it is a sad loss for her. Let her know she and her mother are missed.

Activities Of Daily Living

Make sure Mrs. Reston is dressed in comfortable, soft, loose fitting, and favorite bedclothes. Make sure her linens are clean and smell good. Pay attention to odors and cleanliness to increase her comfort and the comfort of her visitors. Use pillows and padding to help her find several comfortable positions. Every effort should be made to make it easy for Frances to spend time with her mother. Offer comfort foods and drinks. She may eat better if someone sings to her.

Activities

Soothing activities work best. If Mrs. Reston pulls at her covers, perhaps a soft quilt or stuffed animal or doll will comfort her. A radio or audiotape player can be used to play her favorite music or nature or water sounds. Involve a music therapist. Often rhythmic activities will soothe and substitute for repetitive pulling and tugging. Stroking or light massage can be comforting, particularly in combination with pain medication.

Some dying residents are comforted when a family member climbs into bed with them. If Frances is comfortable with this idea, suggest it as a way to ease her mother's passage. Encourage her to talk, sing, pray, or just hold her. Remind her that it will not hurt her mother if she cries.

Environmental Strategies

- Mrs. Reston might be more comfortable in a private room. If this is not possible, her roommate should be encouraged to spend time out of the room, or a movable screen should separate them.
- Soften lights and reduce noise and glare. Place signs over her bed reminding all staff of her personal preferences for positioning, music, or reassuring topics. Frances will appreciate your attempt to individualize her mother's care.

- Bring in bright flowers or position her to view her favorite comfort items or scenery. A lava lamp or something with soft colors and slow motion may have a calming effect.
- Some residents are comforted by visible religious symbols like a rosary or cross.
- Experiment with aromatherapy and a room humidifier.
- Pad the bedrails to prevent bruising and consider a special mattress to increase comfort or reduce skin breakdown.

Tip Checklist

1. Comfort at the end of life includes pain management and a healing presence.
2. Swallowing and choking problems should be addressed with changes in feeding techniques and foods offered.
3. Be available to families at the time of death and in bereavement.

Chapter 4

HELPING FAMILIES ADJUST TO LONG TERM CARE

Today, Mrs. Utley is moving into The Garden, an assisted living facility unit that specializes in caring for people with memory disorders. Her husband and daughter feel guilty about their "failed" efforts to "keep Mom at home where she belongs." Recently, due to her disease, Mrs. Utley has been keeping her husband up all night and frequently leaves the house while he dozes. The last time she wandered off at night, she was gone long enough to become dehydrated and required hospitalization. The doctors told Mr. Utley that his wife was ready for residential care and needed more care than an 85-year-old husband with a bad heart could be expected to provide. Fortunately, their daughter had met with the staff of The Garden before the latest crisis and filled out initial admission forms. Mrs. Utley arrives with her frantic husband and tearful daughter looking uncertain and confused.

How can you ease this difficult transition for Mrs. Utley and her family?

Admission Day: Setting The Stage For A Smooth Transition

Helping families become comfortable with the decision to admit a loved one to a long term care facility begins by focusing attention on the new resident. Reassuring the guilty family may seem like the right first step, but the family primarily is concerned about Mrs. Utley. Therefore, to reassure the family about their placement decision, staff should demonstrate the caring attitude they will provide to Mrs. Utley. To do this, staff should welcome Mrs.

Utley and tell her how nice she looks and how everyone is so pleased that she is here. Keep it brief and simple.

Staff should have asked all relevant questions and filled out forms earlier, because most families are too overwhelmed to answer all of the necessary questions on the day of admission. In addition, having Mrs. Utley's history in advance will make the transition easier, since staff will be able to talk with her about her life and will know some of her favorite foods and activities.

Staff should introduce themselves to Mrs. Utley and her family, show Mrs. Utley staff name tags, and tell her that the staff is here to help her be comfortable. Let her know that this is a good place and that she will like the people here. Also, tell her that her husband has insisted on the very best for her and staff's goal is to live up to his high expectations. Find a private way to let Mr. Utley and his daughter know that a move like this is always hardest on the families that have cared for and done the most for their relative. Staff should tell the family how much their devotion is noticed and admired. Remind them that this is not a hospital and open visiting is their right and is welcomed.

If the family looks sad, ask them if they would like to talk about their feelings or frustrations. If Mrs. Utley becomes mad or suspicious and demands to go home, say, "I know you would rather be home, but I would like you to stay for now. Sometimes we just have to do hard things. I know you would like more choices, but this is the best we can offer for today." Let Mrs. Utley and her family express their sadness and anger, but give them hope that with time they will adjust and feel better about their decision.

Next, staff should show the family to Mrs. Utley's room and encourage the family to sit down and have a drink or a snack together. At this point, staff should begin talking about some of Mrs. Utley's past and current interests. Encourage her family to reassure her that they care about her and will help to make this transition easier. Also, suggest that the family bring items for her room to remind her of happy times in her past, such as favorite photos or books. However, do not rush the family to move everything in or set up the entire room immediately. Recommend that they use the time with Mrs. Utley now to take a walk around The Garden and meet some of the "neighbors." Staff should point out important places like her bathroom and the dining room while reassuring the family that staff will ensure that Mrs. Utley receives all the assistance she needs.

Staff should ask the family if they would like some private time or if they have any questions. Encourage them to take time to get settled. Offer simple choices to Mrs. Utley, such as, "Would you like to see the dining room or the library first?" If Mrs. Utley becomes demanding, reassure her that her requests will be handled immediately. Keep repeating that staff will make sure she settles in comfortably.

Provide the family with written information about routines. Encourage them to call the facility anytime with questions. Even though the move is serious, humor is always a good tonic.

Most people with AD respond well to calm, polite comments without long explanations or excuses. When speaking with Mrs. Utley, keep saying, "We're doing fine, and I know we will get along well." Do not tell her this is "her home now."

If Mr. Utley and his daughter have trouble leaving, suggest that they go run "a few errands" while staff gets to know Mrs. Utley. Encourage them to give her a hug and tell her they will be back. Let them know they are welcome to come back as soon as they can, but that you will help Mrs. Utley while they are busy. Make sure they leave a security object and a favorite piece of clothing behind for Mrs. Utley to wear. In addition, encourage them to call her if they will be "delayed" and tell Mrs. Utley that you will help her call them whenever she needs them. Tell them that staff and Mrs. Utley will be looking forward to seeing them when they return.

Encourage the family to help their relative meet other residents who could become friends. The facility may not be home, but it can become a community. Encourage families to attend Alzheimer's Association or other support group meetings together. The meetings offer opportunities to discuss concerns and frustrations with the disease and to share experiences in a supportive atmosphere.

Setting Expectations

This move may be as disorienting for Mr. Utley as it is for his wife. Many families feel lost when they no longer are required to provide the constant care that has overwhelmed every waking moment. Families need to know that the facility understands their grief, sadness, loss, and guilt. Staff can comfort Mr. Utley by telling him that some residents look and feel better with the structured, predictable routines and abilities-oriented program offered at the facility. Also explain that he may notice that his wife responds better to a staff member than she has to him lately. Keep reminding him that this behavior is normal with this disease.

Importantly, inform families that most people with Alzheimer's have difficulty remembering what is done for them or to them. Mrs. Utley may tell her husband that she is not fed, for example, even though she just ate. Encourage families to check out all resident complaints or accusations, and assure them that you will work with the family to prevent further misunderstandings.

Keeping Families Involved In The Caregiving Process

Family involvement is a key component of compassionate Alzheimer's care. Therefore, encourage the family to attend care planning meetings and stay involved in the resident's care. Ask the family about their priorities and concerns—not all families value the same things. For Mr. Utley, it may be most important to see his wife dressed up each day with makeup and jewelry. His daughter may be more concerned about her mother's food intake. But almost all families want staff to get to know as much about their relative's likes and dislikes and to respect resident wishes to the extent possible.

Staff can also encourage families to join them in solving the mysteries or unknowns in how to work with each resident. Brainstorming can take place during family visits as well as at formal care planning sessions. Staff and family members should tell each other everything they have tried in the past to deal with specific needs or problems of the resident. For instance, if Mrs. Utley refuses to bathe at the facility, she probably refused to bathe at home as well. Strategies used successfully at home can be tried at the facility. If these do not work, staff and family together can come up with other ideas.

Also, let families know that Alzheimer's care is hard and can be frustrating whether it is provided by families or residential care staff. Explain that staff and the family need each other to help provide the best care and most stimulating environment for their loved one. Because of the behavioral and communication deficits associated with AD, families will expect staff to check routinely for signs of potential illness or injury.

Prepare families for the unexpected. For example, daily baths are not common, meals are served in a dining room, and each nurse assistant has a number of residents to care for. Give families opportunities to talk when staff is not rushed—either by setting up special meetings for new families or finding a quiet time of day to speak about issues or concerns.

Visiting Tips

Many families have a difficult time visiting and may become disappointed when the resident does not remember the visit, accuses them of abandonment, or looks sloppy. Families appreciate suggestions for improving the quality of their visits. Facilities with active family visitors are generally seen as more interesting places to work or live. Offer families the following tips and guidelines to make visits positive and enjoyable.

- It's the quality—not the quantity—of visits that makes a difference to residents. Bring something to do together or spend time with other residents and their families. Visit when you are not rushed and do not stay so long that you and the resident are worn out.

- You may not always see the staff you are looking for when you visit. Leave notes for the staff and ask them to leave notes for you about special things that your relative did or needs since your last visit.

- Alternate visits with other family members and friends. Encourage church and social friends to visit at times when the resident is most alert. Invite friends and provide suggestions for activities during their visit.

- Create visiting rituals: Bring a milkshake to share on a hot afternoon, check out the bird feeder or fish tank, visit another resident, or bring a craft project, favorite video, or audiotape to enjoy together.

- Quiet shared moments are just as meaningful as "gab" sessions about current family events. Listening to hymns or saying prayers together, polishing nails, brushing hair, or massaging the resident's hand can promote feelings of togetherness and belonging.

- Use props for reminiscing about the old days. For instance, bring photo albums or scrapbooks, old magazines, sewing patterns, or tools, and talk about them. Sometimes, residents enjoy repeating favorite stories, jokes, poems, or songs.

- Love is portable. You do not have to be present to send your love in a telephone call, a videotape, a letter, or a card. Your loving message may be "delivered" by a friend or relative in your absence or by another resident's family.

Helping Families Cope

Ask the family how you can help meet their needs. You can do this during visits, at care planning conferences, or with a questionnaire sent to the family's home. Start a Family Network: Introduce new families to veterans of nursing facility care. Families of residents who have been at the facility for a long time may be helped themselves in trying to help others. Such efforts can snowball into a family support group. Important discussion topics might include dealing with loss, getting more out of visits and talks with staff, life after placement, and asking for help.

Encourage families who are really distressed to seek counseling from a social worker, pastor, or outside counselor who can listen and reassure them. Start a family resource center in the facility with information about Alzheimer's and nursing facility care. Have each staff member take responsibility for a small group of families. This helps families have their questions answered quickly.

Suggest rituals: Many residents and families have a strong faith and take comfort in rituals that mark changes in one's life. A ritual marking the move to a new home that includes readings, poems, and prayers can ease healing.

Invite families to social events or facility holiday gatherings. Some facilities offer dinners outside the facility for new families to get to know staff in a more neutral setting.

Finally, suggest personally meaningful volunteer opportunities for family members who have the time and interest.

Chapter 5

ENVIRONMENTS THAT ENCOURAGE BELONGING

'When the fog rolls in, I think I'm drowning. I can feel the emptiness inside.'

—Resident with Alzheimer's

Residential care is expected to be homelike, but residents with Alzheimer's—and their families—have very different notions of "home." Everyone wants the place they live to be clean, comfortable, safe, and attractive. Most people with Alzheimer's are comfortable in places where they feel like they belong. That is a real challenge in group living when residents from such different backgrounds come together and may even share a room with a stranger.

People with Alzheimer's have the same need for and right to privacy as other residents. Some people with Alzheimer's, however, get scared when they are alone in their rooms and may need to stay around the staff work area or in other residents' rooms—or even other residents' beds. Other residents may become overwhelmed by so many other people and may retreat to their beds, where they feel more secure. Some people with Alzheimer's were always loners, and others may have always paced or wandered off in search of excitement.

Residents with dementia deserve the choice to be in their rooms or out in public areas and may leave their doors open or closed. At the same time, good facilities create a sense of belonging or community, perhaps through neighborhood units or cottages that share common areas. To succeed in helping residents with Alzheimer's feel like they belong, they need access to a variety of spaces for different purposes.

Special care units (SCUs) traditionally have been secured areas to keep people safe from the hazards of wandering away from the facility. But Alzheimer-friendly environments are actually places that are designed to balance stimulation and retreat options throughout the facility. People with Alzheimer's need interesting places that draw them out of their rooms. They also need small quiet places where they can retreat from too much noise, stimulation, or confusion.

To make the facility's environment AD-friendly, install cues in the environment—tips to help residents know what is around the corner or that they have reached the bathroom. For example, the smell of food might lead to a kitchen area, while a picture of a toilet might remind a resident to use it. Cues can be unit-based, such as guides to common areas, or they can be personal. Pictures of a resident's mother and father with the resident as a child might help a resident find the right room in which to lie down. A crocheted headrest on a favorite chair may help a resident recognize that chair as her own. Hanging clothes in the closet in the order that they will be put on may be just the cue needed to help the resident dress herself. A favorite old hat or a familiar sign hung on the door to a man's room may help him find his room.

Sensory cues, such as the smell of baking, will draw residents to a cooking activity. The sounds of hammering may bring out curiosity and interest for other residents. Piano music may draw people to a social activity in the living room, or a church bell may be sounded when chapel services are about to begin. Some facilities have experimented with murals of street scenes from the past or scenes of people dressed in 1920s clothing all walking in the same direction to encourage movement that way.

To discourage residents from entering areas that are off limits, simple stop signs may cue residents to turn away from exit doors. An old desk with lots of mail and items to sort may create a stop along the way for hallway walkers. Park benches and plants in hall alcoves may encourage residents to stop, rest, and chat with other residents. A children's playground visible from indoors may draw reluctant residents outdoors to a tree-enclosed safe outdoor area. Seasonal items indoors or outdoors may remind residents of holidays, the weather outside, or a time of year that they especially enjoyed.

Creating Special Neighborhoods

Some residential care and nursing facilities are moving toward scaled-down units that look more like single-family homes. These smaller living units encourage friendships among staff and residents. They also make sense to Alzheimer's residents and make it easier for staff to provide discrete surveillance and supervision. Most of these model units are small units of larger facilities that provide plenty of places to explore safely without exiting unnoticed.

Residents live in small, private bedrooms; they share a common small kitchen, eating, and living area; and often have a secured front porch, rooftop porch, or outdoor shaded area that draws people outside. Key elements of these smaller residential groupings are that the private bedroom areas are grouped away from public areas, providing minimal distractions from noise and noncare staff; there is good visual access from bedrooms to common areas; and there are safe indoor and outdoor paths for exploring. Familiar activities of daily living take place in recognizable spaces. Larger living rooms can be separated for two small-group activities with decorative dividers or potted plants.

Other facilities have opened up previously off-limits areas, such as kitchens, dining rooms, and laundry rooms to people with Alzheimer's. Many people with Alzheimer's will feel at home setting or clearing a table, having coffee with staff at a kitchen table, or in a small laundry area where they can sort and fold clothes, iron towels on a cool setting, or chat. All these normal, everyday activities encourage socializing among residents and with staff.

Still other facilities create small libraries, craft or work rooms, card rooms, or music rooms to encourage activities outside the scheduled large-group activity programs. Many facilities try to balance sensory overload with enough sensory stimulation by removing clutter, providing touchable art and interesting fabric coverings, and limiting the noise of alarms and televisions. Because of unique visual issues of people with Alzheimer's—such as problems with depth perception, color discrimination, contrast sensitivity, and the ability to ignore visual distractions—environmental designers recommend reducing glare, creating partitions with cloth to block confusing things from view, increasing contrast in colors to highlight thresholds, and increasing exposure to bright light. Extra light and contrasting colors also can highlight obstacles, cues, and grab bars.

Larger facilities may have an ice cream bar or coffee shop open certain hours to create new opportunities for socializing. Large dining rooms can be used in off-hours for visiting, card games, and special activities. One facility created an old-fashioned bank teller's window that was staffed certain hours to give Alzheimer's residents the chance to mimic doing their banking as they always did. These are just a few ways to adapt existing environments to make them seem more normal and familiar to people with Alzheimer's.

One large facility with an on-site preschool successfully partnered the program with residents who had Alzheimer's by having them help the children with learning activities. These preschoolers also went for daily rides on a big wagon through the facility to greet their resident friends and "teachers." The children's outdoor play area was visible from resident rooms and prompted lots of conversations about which children belonged to which staff members.

Many facilities also experiment with exercise rooms that look more like health clubs than physical therapy rooms. Residents can safely use the exercise equipment whenever it is available and if they are interested. Adapted work environments also are a good idea. With the right space, residents can work in small groups on volunteer projects. Some creative facilities have found room for old model cars that can be safely entered, tinkered with, and used for reminiscing about first road trips.

On a smaller scale, bedrooms, bathrooms, and toilet facilities can be scaled down to look more inviting. Plants and decorative tile, towel heaters, soft music, or plush terry robes can soften bathing rooms and reduce the echo from hard surfaces. Skylights can be used indoors to create a more open feeling. Outdoor areas can be made more inviting with comfortable seating, paths that curve and do not just go in a circle, and healing or therapeutic gardens. These gardens may have seating for family groups, private visiting, and relaxing areas; shaded resting areas; safe plant materials for four seasons of sensory stimulation; smooth, safe walking surfaces; and plantings in containers at ground and raised levels. Simple birdbaths and umbrella tables with chairs can add interest to an outdoor area. Old-time boardwalk music could be piped in.

It is wise to consider regional traditions in adapting environments for people with Alzheimer's. In some regions, it may be more important to have a chapel in the facility than a library. Facilities in regions with mild weather year-round have more of an incentive to invest in elaborate outdoor areas than do facilities with harsh winters. People from large cities will expect city environments. One facility in New Mexico was built of adobe with arched doorways and fireplaces. Coastal communities may expect more fishing or beach-like areas or designs. Many facilities adapt to residents' preferences and change the use of spaces to fit the needs of long-stay residents. At a minimum, all facilities try to personalize the sleeping space of Alzheimer residents to help them recognize their room as different from everyone else's.

Environmental Tips

- Physical features make programming and relationships thrive, but no design features will make up for inadequate programming or an impersonal human and social environment.
- Personalize bedrooms even if shared. Use shelves, wide window ledges, and flat furniture tops to display mementos. Personalize entrances to resident rooms.
- Brighten light levels and use night lights.
- Use sheer curtains on windows and low-gloss floor wax to reduce glare.
- Minimize the visibility of alarms and carts.
- Place sturdy items next to the path from the bed to the toilet to help provide stability to residents.
- Use simple signs at eye level with bright contrasting colors for residents. Minimize staff signs.
- Use high-color contrast among dishes, tablecloths, and placemats at meals.
- Use aromas (like percolating coffee) to cue mealtimes or dining areas.
- Play tapes of bird sounds for residents who have trouble getting going in the morning.
- To disguise an exit, paint it the same color as the wall, or put black tape across the floor in front of the door.
- Keep temperatures warm.
- Use large door handles.
- Create paths that encourage strolling.
- Create workstations that have interesting, safe articles for individual or group use, such as desks with catalogues, files, and papers or a digging plot.
- Use small clusters of seating to view outside or activity areas.
- Provide chairs with arms that extend to the front edge of the seat.
- Provide seating along hallways, outdoor paths, and at entrances, with chairs at right angles.
- Individualize music preferences with audio headsets, tape players,

or radios.

- Use of textures and sound-absorbing materials like wall hangings in public areas adds warmth, richness, and interest. Create areas that draw people in and encourage them to reach and touch objects.
- Bright, contrasting colors—such as reds and yellows—should accent an overall neutral color scheme. Too many bright colors and graphics can overwhelm and overstimulate residents with AD.
- A sense of humor, tolerance for confusion, and a sense of fun should be conveyed by each staff member. It lightens up the atmosphere.
- Encourage residents to dress up if they like or to dress in their cultural, ethnic, or personal style.

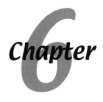

Chapter 6

WHAT TO DO IF YOU ARE HAVING A ROUGH DAY

Caring for residents with Alzheimer's is stressful—just ask their families or any caregiver. It is difficult caring for people who do not recognize their need for care or appreciate efforts on their behalf. Residents thrive on predictable routines, but staff may long for a change of pace or more surprises than just the unpredictable behaviors of the residents.

It is exhausting to have to think, plan, prevent, and respond all day to so many residents who cannot accomplish much for themselves. It also is upsetting to become attached to people who deteriorate despite your best efforts. Watching sad, painful visits with relatives who mourn the loss of "the mother I once knew" also hurts. Families may have little energy for staff because they, too, are emotionally caught up with their loved one.

Upbeat staff develop a tolerance for confusion or strange behavior and hold tight to a sense of humor. Some individuals bring this to their work while others develop it in response to this kind of work. But it is hard to give all the time if you aren't getting something back. Some facilities recognize staff needs and make time for staff support groups, or they send valued staff to conferences or conventions outside the facility. Facilities pay attention to morale by remembering and celebrating staff birthdays, wedding showers, or other personal events. Some creative facilities have parties or contests that bring in the staff's families as well as residents and their families. Some staff just develop friendships on their own that help them handle the stress.

But what if you're having a bad day or week and you need a way to feel more like your better self again? Try these tips and add your own:

- Cut yourself some slack. No one is perfect or patient 100 percent of the time. Decide that tomorrow will be better.
- You can change your actions and reactions to stress. Take slow, deep breaths.
- Count your blessings. Use your faith or belief for extra strength. Remind yourself of the good parts of each day or what's good in your life.
- Find a quiet hideout at work, at home, or in your head—a place, view, picture, fountain, plant, tree, or memory that calms and soothes your spirit or makes you smile.
- Give friends pats on the back if they do something nice. They will do the same for you when you need it.
- A change of pace helps. If you cannot change your work routine, change your routines at home, or simply change your route to work.
- Use your creativity. Do not let an old hobby or craft project sit in the closet.
- Rediscover your sense of humor. Remember: there is a thin line between what's really tasteless and what's really funny.
- Pay attention to what is fun for you. Is it playing with the dog, sports, cooking, or playing with your kids?
- Say "no" and mean it if you are at your limit. Too much work is bad for the soul.
- Get enough sleep, good food, and exercise.
- Stay involved in groups you enjoy. Drop the rest.
- Preserve real friendships.
- Say, "I will not let this get to me. I will go with the flow."
- Never lose sight of your big dreams; they make life seem bigger.

APPENDICES

APPENDIX A

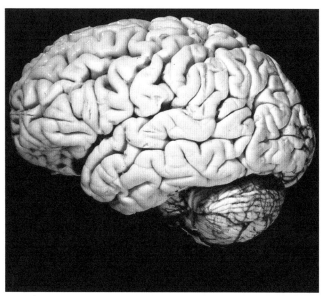

Normal Brain
vs.
Alzheimer's Brain

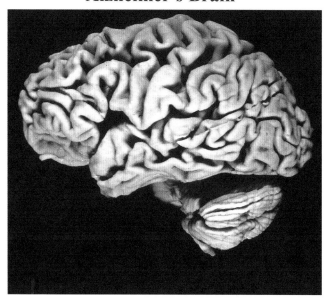

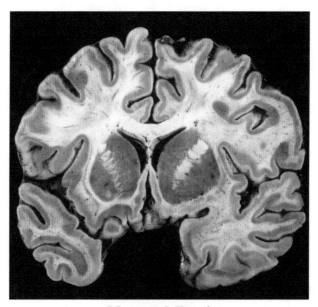

Normal Brain
vs.
Alzheimer's Brain

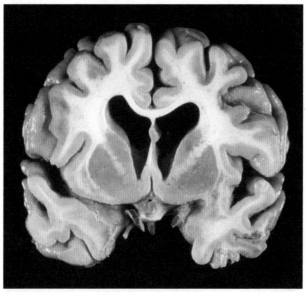

ides courtesy of Dr. Christine Hulette, Neuropathologist, Bryan Alzheimer's Disease Research Center, Duke University Medical Center.

APPENDIX B

CHARACTERISTICS OF ALZHEIMER'S DISEASE

ALZHEIMER'S IS:

- A diagnosable brain disease
- The most common form of dementia
- Progressive—it gets worse over time
- More than memory loss
- A common disorder among residents of assisted living and nursing facilities
- Variable in symptoms and duration

ALZHEIMER'S DISEASE IS NOT:

- Normal aging or amnesia
- Limited to people over 65 or to a specific race, religion, ethnic, or educational group
- Diagnosed by a single blood test or X-ray
- Mental retardation
- A character flaw or laziness
- Contagious
- Currently preventable or curable

COMMON CHANGES IN MILD ALZHEIMER'S

- Loses spark or zest for life—does not start anything.
- Loses recent memory without a change in appearance or casual conversation.
- Loses judgment about money.
- Has difficulty with new learning and making new memories.
- Has trouble finding words—may substitute or make up words that sound like or mean something like the forgotten word.
- May stop talking to avoid making mistakes.
- Has shorter attention span and less motivation to stay with an activity.
- Easily loses way going to familiar places.
- Resists change or new things.
- Has trouble organizing and thinking logically.
- Asks repetitive questions.
- Withdraws, loses interest, is irritable, not as sensitive to other's feelings, uncharacteristically angry when frustrated or tired.
- Won't make decisions—"I'll have what she is having."
- Takes longer to do routine chores and becomes upset if rushed or if something unexpected happens.
- Forgets to pay, pays too much, or forgets how to pay—may hand the check-out person a wallet instead of the correct amount of money.
- Forgets to eat, eats only one kind of food, or eats constantly.
- Loses or misplaces things by hiding them in odd places or forgets where things go, such as putting clothes in the dishwasher.
- Constantly checks, searches, or hoards things of no value.

COMMON CHANGES IN MODERATE ALZHEIMER'S

- Changes in behavior, concern for appearance, hygiene, and sleep become more noticeable.
- Mixes up identity of people, such as thinking a son is a brother or that a wife is a stranger.
- Poor judgment creates safety issues when left alone: may wander and risk exposure, poisoning, falls, self-neglect, or exploitation.
- Has trouble recognizing familiar people and own objects: may take things that belong to others.
- Continuously repeats stories, favorite words, statements, or motions like tearing tissues.
- Has restless, repetitive movements in late afternoon or evening—pacing, trying doorknobs, fingering draperies.
- Cannot organize thoughts or follow logical explanations.
- Has trouble following written notes or completing tasks.
- Makes up stories to fill in gaps in memory. Might say, "Mama will come for me when she gets off work."
- May be able to read but cannot formulate the correct response to a written request.
- May accuse, threaten, curse, fidget, or behave inappropriately, such as kicking, hitting, biting, screaming, or grabbing at nurse assistants.
- May become sloppy or forget manners.
- May see, hear, smell, or taste things that are not there.
- May accuse spouse of an affair or staff or family of stealing.
- Naps frequently or awakens at night believing it is time to go to work.
- Has more difficulty positioning the body to use the toilet or sit in a chair.
- May think mirror image is following him or television story is happening to her.
- Needs help finding the toilet, using the shower, remembering to drink, and dressing for the weather or occasion.

- Exhibits inappropriate sexual behavior, such as mistaking staff or another resident for a spouse.
- Forgets what is private behavior, and may disrobe or masturbate in public.

COMMON CHANGES IN SEVERE ALZHEIMER'S

- Doesn't recognize self or close family.
- Speaks in gibberish, is mute, or is difficult to understand.
- May refuse to eat, chokes, or forgets to swallow.
- May repetitively cry out, pat, or touch everything.
- Loses control of bowel and bladder.
- Loses weight and skin becomes thin and tears easily.
- May look uncomfortable or cry out when transferred or touched.
- Forgets how to walk or is too unsteady or weak to stand alone.
- May have seizures, frequent infections, falls.
- May groan, scream, or mumble loudly.
- Sleeps more.
- Needs total assistance for all activities of daily living.

APPENDIX C

REFERENCES

• For help: Contact an Alzheimer's Association chapter. Ask for the chapter newsletter and show it to families who may not know about this source of help.

Alzheimer's Association
919 N. Michigan Ave., Suite 1100
Chicago, IL 60611-1676
TOLL FREE: 800-272-3900
Web site: http://www.alz.org
Green-Field Library/Reference:
312-335-9602

• Build a library of AD materials; your Alzheimer's Association chapter can make suggestions.

• Sponsor a public awareness/fund raising event like an Alzheimer's Association Memory Walk with experts, materials, and even celebrities.

• Talk with the families of Alzheimer's residents in your facility. Many have become experts on AD and caring techniques and would love to learn from you as well. Encourage their participation in in-service presentations.

• Alzheimer's Association publications
(1997) *Key Elements of Dementia Care* (PF 3082)
(1995) *Solving Bathing Problems* (Book and video; ED 2602)
(1995) *Activity Programming for Persons with Dementia: A Sourcebook* (PF 3062)
(2000) *Alzheimer's Videos: An Annotated Guide* (LIB 5062)

Order Toll Free/Customer Service: 800-223-4405;
fax: 877-356-9119; email: alz@pbd.com
Alzheimer's Association, PO Box 930408, Atlanta, GA 31193-0408

TO LEARN MORE:

Alzheimer's Disease Education and Referral Center (ADEAR)
PO Box 8250
Silver Spring, MD 20907-8250
Toll Free: 800-438-4380
http://www.alzheimers.org
Excellent training materials for care staff.

American Therapeutic Recreation Association: 1414 Prince Street, Suite 204, Alexandria, VA 22314; 703-683-9420; www.atra-tr.org

American Music Therapy Association: 8455 Colesville Rd., Suite 1000, Silver Spring, MD 20910; 301-589-3300; e-mail: info@musictherapy.org; Web site: www.musictherapy.org.

National Association of Activity Professionals: PO Box 5530, Sevierville, TN 37865; 423-429-9914; e-mail: THENAAP@aol.com.

Alzheimer's Care Quarterly. Carol Bowlby Sifton, Editor. Quarterly journal from Aspen Publishers; www.aspenpublishers.com/journals/acq; 800-638-8437.

Andresen, Gayle (1995) *Caring for People with Alzheimer's Disease: A Training Manual for Direct Care Providers*. Baltimore, MD: Health Professions Press.

Bell, V. and Troxel, D. (1997) *The Best Friends Approach to Alzheimer's Care*. Baltimore, MD: Health Professions Press.

Bell, V. and Troxel, D. (2000) *The Best Friends Staff: Building A Culture of Care in Alzheimer's Programs*. Baltimore, MD: Health Professions Press.

Ballard, E., Gwyther, L. and Toal, T.P. (2000). *Pressure Points: Alzheimer's and Anger*. Duke Family Support Program, Box 3600 DUMC, Durham, NC 27710; 919-660-7510.

Dyer, L. (1996) *In a Tangled Wood*. Dallas, TX: Southern Methodist University Press (paperback). A daughter's view of an Alzheimer's special care unit.

Gwyther, L.P. (1995) *You Are One of Us: Successful Clergy/Church Connections to Alzheimer's Families*. $4 prepaid to Duke Family Support Program, Box 3600, DUMC, Durham, NC 27710.

Hellen, Carly R. (Second Edition, 1998) *Alzheimer's Disease: Activity-Focused Care*. Boston, MA: Butterworth Heineman. http://www.bh.com.

Henderson, C.S. (1998) *Partial View*. Dallas, TX: Southern Methodist University Press (paperback). A pictorial essay of what it is like to have Alzheimer's by a historian with advanced Alzheimer's disease.

Kaplan, M. and Hoffman, S. (1998) *Behaviors in Dementia: Best Practice for Successful Management*. Baltimore, MD: Health Professions Press.

Lawton, M. Powell and Rubinstein, Robert L., Editors.(2000) *Interventions in Dementia Care: Toward Improving Quality of Life*. New York, NY: Springer Publishing.

Nursing Assistant Monthly, Special Issue on Dementia Care, July/August 1999, Vol. 5, No. 7: Frontline Publishing, 800-348-0605.

Speaking From Experience: *Nursing Assistants Share Their Knowledge of Dementia Care* (1997). Cobble Hill Health Center,

Inc. 380 Henry St., Brooklyn, NY, 11201; 718-852-6789, fax 718-852-5673, or e-mail nk105@columbia.edu.

Rader, J. (1995) *Individualized Dementia Care: Creative, Compassionate Approaches.* New York, NY: Springer Publishing.

Smith, Marianne and Buckwalter, Kathleen C. (1998) *Choice and Challenge: Caring for Aggressive Older Adults Across Care Settings.* Video and printed materials available from Terra Nova Films, Chicago, IL; 800-779-8491; email http://www.terranova.org. See other videos on Alzheimer's facility care from Terra Nova: "A Day in the Life of Nancy Moore" (1990), "Dealing with Physical Aggression in Caregiving: Non-Physical and Physical Interventions" (2000).

Fanlight Productions, "Dress Him While He Walks," (1995), 800-937-4113, www.fanlight.com.

Volicer, L. and Bloom-Charette, L., Editors. (1999) *Enhancing the Quality of Life in Advanced Dementia.* Philadelphia, PA: Brunner/Mazel; 215-625-8900.

Zgola, J.M. (1999) *Care That Works: A Relationship Approach to Persons with Dementia.* Baltimore, MD: The Johns Hopkins University Press; www.press.jhu.edu